What people a

Healthy Fashion

I think it's a wonderfully fresh approach to fashion and I applaud the author's attempt to open a whole new paradigm here.

Dreamweaver, founder/owner of Sapien Medicine, Enlightened States

The importance of fashion should not be underestimated. Fashion is not only a reflection of an individual, but also of a culture, of a society, and the values that people hold dear; fashion has the power to shape individuals and collective groups. Think of the varied costumes on the stage of life; think about the power of military or medical uniforms. Fashion, and the materials from which our clothing is created, immediately advertises (truly or falsely) who we are, what we aspire to, and our pretenses. How you present yourself to the external world has the power to shape your inner spiritual being – we become the fashion we display. With such thoughts in mind, close consideration of the concepts of *Healthy Fashion* should be imperative for anyone interested in the subject.

Robert M. Schoch, PhD, geologist and author of *Forgotten Civilization*

What Alyssa writes really resonated with me. I have long believed, as she has, that plant-based materials should comprise the bulk of our wardrobes. Given that many top designers are cutting fur from their collections, and that hemp is making a comeback, I feel that her ideas about the relationship between humans, plants and fashion are highly prescient.

Chere Di Boscio, founder/owner of *Eluxe Magazine*

2020 is the beginning of heightened Consciousness on Earth, and it is certainly the "Time for Healthy Fashion." Alyssa combines fashion with spirit. Many new modes of healing have made their debut in the last few years, such as the use of Color and Sound Therapy and Sacred Geometries. Highly evolved civilizations wear only brightly colored clothing made of natural fibers and hemp. Our cells are "Alive" and sense and feel the color and fabric of clothing against our skin. Alyssa has certainly tuned into the Creator Frequency, and I highly recommend her book *Healthy Fashion*.

Dianne Robbins, author of *Messages from the Hollow Earth*

A book that passionately and comprehensively faces the issue of unhealthy fashion, and how it affects humans' body and soul. Healthy fashion means healthy people, a great message for the future.

Mikel Guido Dolci, founder and CEO of GreenFashionWeek

Healthy Fashion

The Deeper Truths

Healthy Fashion

The Deeper Truths

Alyssa Couture

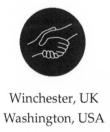

Winchester, UK
Washington, USA

JOHN HUNT PUBLISHING

First published by Ayni Books, 2021
Ayni Books is an imprint of John Hunt Publishing Ltd., No. 3 East Street, Alresford
Hampshire SO24 9EE, UK
office@jhpbooks.com
www.johnhuntpublishing.com
www.ayni-books.com

For distributor details and how to order please visit the 'Ordering' section on our website.

Design: Stuart Davies

UK: Printed and bound by CPI Group (UK) Ltd, Croydon, CR0 4YY
Printed in North America by CPI GPS partners

We operate a distinctive and ethical publishing philosophy in all areas of our business, from our global network of authors to production and worldwide distribution.

Contents

.

"Willpower alone makes chaos; realization alone is dead. Combine both and you have a powerful, creative flame from the Universe."
Hanna Kroeger

Introduction: About *Healthy Fashion*

Fashion for health; a new approach

Healthy Fashion is a new model of modern, fresh, and high fashion designed for human health. Fashion for health is a new approach to fashion that awakens the soul and spirit. It is apparel used as an integrative tool and as an alternative medicine. When healthy fashion is worn, we become healthy fashion practitioners.

We are living during an exciting time. It is the perfect time to introduce concepts of fashion for health. Fashion for health is an enlightening pursuit for this modern era. We are in a time of a spiritual and planetary awakening, and the fashion industry is in a bit of a transition right now. Fashion for health is being produced and promoted in a gradual progression, in pursuit of healing the mind, body, and spirit.

The main topics in *Healthy Fashion*

• **Fashion deemed medicinal** *Healthy Fashion* establishes an alternative, modern approach to clothing: fashion deemed medicinal. Fashion becomes medicinal when it treats the body therapeutically and multidimensionally. Multidimensional fashion is fashion for physical, mental, emotional, energetic, and spiritual health. Fashion, to cure the ails of the body, is an important part of dress that will bring the Earth and humans back into balance.

• **Plant-based fabrics** Plant-based clothing is the future of fashion. Plant-based fabrics are the ultimate to wear for health and wellbeing. The connection we have with plants is ancient. Dressing in plant-based fashion is a sacred, healing art. From aquatic plants, to wild weeds, to farm-cultivated crops; a wide

1

range and an assortment of plants to be produced into fabrics is the future of fashion. Fashion made from nature is beneficial for the complete healing of the body's suffering and unnatural conditions.

• **Universal fashion:** Universal fashion merges cultures together, in pursuit of bringing fashion into a state of worldwide equilibrium. It eliminates the discriminating conflicts in fashion that create segregation and disconnection. It celebrates human diversity and human uniqueness combined, inducing the wisdom of fashion to shine through. Universal fashion transcends fashion stereotypes that tend to segregate people, and it promotes the fashion archetype model which is a person's individual, unique self, expressed through their fashion. Archetype fashion is personal style being expressed on the soul level.

• **Unhealthy fashion:** Unhealthy fashion is explained in the book, in order to decipher what is and what is not healthy to wear. Unhealthy fashion is void of spirit and based on an unhealthy, ego-based type of fulfillment. Negative fashion has an impure vibration that does not support the body. Additionally, synthetic fabrics like polyester, nylon and acrylic are not the healthiest, because they are not of similar chemical composition to that of the human body. They suppress the body because they are unbreathable. The toxic chemicals used to make the fabrics are creating hazardous effects. Yet, most of us still wear synthetic, petroleum-based fabrics, and it is OK to wear them. It's all about transition.

Specific ways fashion can heal the five bodies that are addressed in *Healthy Fashion*:
• **Physically:** The capabilities of plant-based fabrics and their health benefits that physically support the body are addressed

in this book. The pros and advantages of healthy, natural, plant-based fabrics, versus the cons and disadvantages of petroleum-based and animal-based fabrics are included in the book.

• **Mentally:** Less fashion hierarchy, and more balanced social dynamics in fashion will help create a healthier fashion perception. Creating more unity across the world through fashion proves to be the most beneficial for mental health. In the book, I explain the fashion archetype model: fashion inspired by the Jungian Archetypes, which creates consciousness and enlightenment for the wearer and passerby. Negative, programmed, patterns occur when we perceive fashion by their stereotype.

• **Emotionally/Energetically:** The emotional body and the energy body are both very much affected by fashion. Choosing fashion that celebrates and embraces human emotions will support the wearer. I include the ways apparel can support positive emotions, and release negative energy and toxic emotions.

• **Spiritually:** In *Healthy Fashion*, I talk about how we can use fashion as a spiritual channel to be in higher realms and higher states of existence. Bringing the divine into the fashion picture is a part of our spiritual awakening and of our Earth's planetary awakening. Choosing fashions that celebrate the soul and spirit eliminates fashion that feeds the false ego and any negative influences.

Immediate ways we can be practitioners of healthy fashion:
• Wearing ergonomic clothing that makes us feel happy and comfortable.
• Wearing plant-based fabrics like linen, cotton, and hemp

directly next to the body, and as a part of the first layer of an outfit. Synthetic fiber garments should ultimately be worn as the second or preferably the third layer of an outfit. They need to fit loosely on the body, to maintain breathability.

• We need to strengthen the connection we have with our clothing. We can choose outfits that evoke our own "soul presence." It is the wisdom, spirit, and art of fashion that helps strengthen our "soul presence." Clothing that is a natural extension of one's individuality, and clothing that is in communion with the environment and existence supports confidence and self-esteem.

What inspired me to write *Healthy Fashion*?

I noticed a general emptiness and void in fashion, and a lack of fashion for health. As well, I have spent a number of years developing new, interesting, artistic, philosophical and science-based concepts of fashion for health. This inspired me to write a book on fresh, modern fashion for the mind, body, and spirit.

Healthy fashion for the future

Healthy Fashion creates new heights for the mind, body, and soul. It describes new ways fashion can be used as an alternative medicine and healing treatment for the body. It operates as a complete, comprehensive method and practice of advanced fashion remedies. It delivers a fresh take on fashion's effects on the intricate, complex human condition. Healthy fashion is a lifestyle opportunity, that explores the deeper realms of fashion that ignite purpose, value, and virtue.

Healthy Fashion is presented in a digestible way. Its big picture delves into the inner workings of all things fashion, encompassing a generous scope of fashion with all its vastness entailed. Readers are given a multifaceted approach as it communicates a comprehensive set of values, ideas, and vision.

Covering a lot of ground, it identifies with and distinguishes the complexity of the human condition in relation to fashion. *Healthy Fashion* is a forward-thinking book that tunes into a modern lifestyle. Fashion as modern medicine is a relatively new concept, an advanced approach. It taps into the potential of what fashion is and can become. It is made to empower, inspire, and create new dimensions for fashion. It is also made to create futuristic, modern modes of thinking. This book certainly broadens perspective, making fashion work to make a person feel and look beautiful.

For the fashion consumer, fashion professional, and for fashion people in general, this easy-to-use manual conjures positive moves to make every wardrobe and every fashion business a healthy one. *Healthy Fashion* is suited for people interested in fashion with a purpose. It's for those who would like to create a grounded foundation and connection to the deeper truths of fashion. It explains how fashion made medicinal can be sought after and accessible to all.

The undertaking of my ideas, concepts, and research presented here are fused together as a response to the great fashion evolution. A full evaluation of fashion is needed, in order to make it a health practice, and it's carried through in this book. When the human/fashion connection is utilized in a practical as well as new-dimensional way, the health properties of fashion take effect. When these realized fashion efforts are addressed, and taken into account, full-body healing will occur.

There is an awakening happening on planet Earth. It's initiating the need for more conscious fashion. Conscious fashion is representative, effective, and in support of global evolution for a healthier planet. There's a need for wholesomeness in all industry fields and it's gradually happening. Whether it be more grounding and balanced cinema, spiritual music, green transportation, healing foods, or healthier fashions, the list goes on.

Fashion can be a supernatural, multidimensional force in our lives, instilling a heightened sense of connection to the planet we belong to. Fashion as a medical initiative will move humanity into a spiritual awakening. Fashion is, and can further be, an alternative health practice contributing to the modern processes of planetary evolution. As a holistic, natural tool, expressing itself on multidimensional levels, it honors all species and the environment.

Healthy Fashion provides an opportunity to bring about a new healthy fashion consciousness. It explores and harnesses the power of fashion used as a tool and channel for various medical needs. Disease is running rampant. There's a lack of attention being put towards fashion psychology, ergonomic fashion, cosmetic fashion fabrics, and other ways to better utilize fashion for health. Overall, fashion in harmony with humans brings fashion, design, and style to new heights.

The fashion concepts presented in *Healthy Fashion* pertaining to philosophy, sociology, and psychology are a fashion journey and a fashion experience. The fashion concepts and methods in *Healthy Fashion* offer a comprehensive, desirable fashion for health. The many tributes *Heathy Fashion* yields are all taken into account and holistically work in congregation for the main goal: a healthy mind, body, and spirit.

The fashion concepts I developed form the basis of *Healthy Fashion*. Major themes that bring about fashion's evolution are included in the book. It's a culmination of my research, experience, and interests all interconnecting in pursuit of fashion deemed medicinal.

Fashion for health is a progressive under-the-radar concept, an untapped field of study. There is great worth to assert fashion as a medical initiative, yet it is not yet pronounced, compared to current, generic fashion standards. What is currently available does not lend enough pursuit of fashion for our medical and therapeutic-based needs. When we become more naturally attuned to favor fashion as a necessary health practice, it will be produced and widely accessible across the globe.

The health of the human body through fashion is a matter that needs to be ushered into this industry, among other industries, and confronted as a priority. It is an ideal solution, relatable and reachable to everyone. *Healthy Fashion* gives an insider view on how this can be attainable for both fashion consumers and fashion businesses.

There's a void in fashion that prevents fashion for health from being discovered and actualized.

Healthy fashion unconditionally offers much more than what is being presented, keeping the fashion industry unevolved, and it keeps it from its full potential. Like the ocean which remains only 5% explored, we have only explored merely a few plant-based fabrics and very few plant-based dyes on the commercial level of production.

Fashion for health is brought about through a holistic approach. Our basic needs for natural, medicinal apparel are very much a part of a holistic model. True healing potential of medicinal fashion occurs when all of its positive implications are recognized and expressed. Healthy fashion is built as a centering role for healing everyone's lives.

Healthy fashion is about being comfortable in clothing in the present moment. The prime goal is to be most comfortable. Being comfortable gives immediate, positive health effects that naturally include long-term positive health effects.

Healthy fashion can be in effect in a manner of minutes when a person puts on a comfortable cotton or linen ensemble from their wardrobe. Uncomfortable clothing reduces the quality of life. It's a waste of time and energy. If the body experiences even slight discomfort, it is a negative ailment. An ill person is generally uncomfortable. Comfortable clothing can naturally ease discomfort, in general. All the aspects that make up a healthy fashion can do even more. It's better living when fashion for health is the desire.

There's a depth of wisdom in *Healthy Fashion*. It engages aspects of fashion that go below the surface of fashion aesthetics, and engages aspects that move beyond the basic function and performance properties of dress. The gift that fashion is and what it will become in future generations will come to fruition when therapeutic fashion is broadcast on deeper, more advanced levels.

Fashion is typically used as a maintenance and beautification activity, not commonly used as a health practice. Not everyone consciously perceives fashion as a healing modality, yet it's a bit of an unspoken rule. This book offers an opportunity to address, recognize, and enhance unspoken yet already practiced fashion remedies, as well as the fashion remedies that are unheard of and not readily practiced. Much of fashion today already improves lives and performs healing, but more substantial improvements and developments in the fashion industry need to be made.

There are many healing fashion modalities actively used, yet they are not discovered on a mass scale. Neither are they used at the depth and scope for their full, beneficial use. It is a matter of creating fashion as a health practice and upgrading the standards placed on fashion for a much grander level of healing to occur.

The lack of healthy fashion, and the lack of fashion perceived and advertised as a healing modality, is partly caused by the levels of human conditioning, and also by a lack of attentiveness to unhealthy fashion's ill effects. Neither are there enough questions or observations on the depth and degree of how negative or positive fashion can be to one's life. Studies prove that the healing components of fashion made medicinal substantially induce purification and recovery for the body, mind, and spirit.

Healthy Fashion is both scientific and spiritually theoretical. There is a spiritual form of intelligence in fashion. One fundamental aspect of healthy fashion is the therapeutic function of spiritual consciousness in apparel. Additionally, the scientifically proven, factual reasons for how fashion can medicinally treat the body are included in the book.

Fashion is fun, but in many ways, it is very serious. An unconventional theory I find missing is that unhealthy fashion is rooted in social, economic, and environmental concerns. Whether it is a matter of a textile manufacturer's poor waste disposal systems, toxic fabrics, fashion pollution, genetically engineered crops, or the socio-economic concerns behind fashion, they all play a role in human health issues and Earth's imbalance. People have become much more aware of these critical issues at hand, and the major conductor that will eliminate many of them is the production and distribution of plant-based fashion.

Unhealthy fashion produces a negative impact on the mass level, creating a complexity turned complicated. As the planet is affected, human health is affected. *Healthy Fashion* reveals the fashion industry's recurring, historical issues of unhealthy fashion that are currently affecting the world. This is to inform readers about unbeneficial fashion for their own discernment and awareness. In part 2, "Unhealthy Fashion," it creates a case against unhealthy fashion. In part 3, "The Plant-based Fashion Guide," it introduces a plan to recover from fashion gone rogue, presenting optimal fashion solutions to fix it, and transcend its negative force of pattern.

To date, the sustainable fashion market is the most evolved. It is a niche, minority market compared to mainstream fashion, yet it's expanding. The two major sectors of the industry—eco/sustainable fashion and commercial/conventional fashion—

have conflicting paths. Fast fashion, mainstream fashion, sustainable fashion, and healthy fashion, all of these market sectors of the industry are inevitably going to merge as the planet evolves.

When both sustainable and commercial fashion industries produce more therapeutic clothing, this will rapidly reduce and dismantle negative states of fashion. The conflicts between eco fashion and conventional fashion will naturally be transcended through healthy fashion strategies. The industry, as a whole, needs to largely fill this gap and void by producing healthy fashion, and make the priority of health-fortifying apparel emerge.

The current demand for healthy fashion is not operating for its full beneficial use. This is changing because it's a scalable, marketable product and a field of study to be pursued most vigorously. The industry needs to move past conventional fashion and eco fashion, and bring about healthy fashion to eliminate disease. This will administer an expansive, soul-defining purpose of fashion.

Realistically, synthetic fabrics are a main contributor of unhealthy fashion. Ultimately, society's dependence on artificial, petroleum-based fabrics suppresses the body's wellbeing. There is scientific proof that they create unnecessary toxicity and stress on the body. It's possible to get away from synthetic fabrics and produce plant-based fabrics predominantly. However, there are steps to take to make this happen, because it's not only a matter of choice, it's what's available on the market for the consumer.

Our synthetic fabric dependence is primarily due to lack of technology towards the production of plant-based fabrics. The resources are available, but they are not nearly all tapped. However, there's a new demand rising for medicinal, plant-based fabrics that will bring Earth back into balance socially, economically, and environmentally.

In part 1, I advocate the use of what I term "plant-tech" fashion as the future of plant-based fabric technology. It does not imply the whole world wears cotton and that's that. Cotton is the dominant plant-based fabric. Unfortunately, cotton is one of the only plant-based fabrics mass-produced, and is predominantly genetically modified. Cotton is essential, it works, but it cannot contend with the need for more plant fiber variations that are currently in smaller-end production or not yet readily known. These plant fiber varieties offer medicinal value that we've only just begun to tap into.

There's an exciting world of opportunity and interest towards the cultivation of plant-based textiles and dyes, and apparel design to be made available. Some lesser-known plant-based fabrics are in production but they are not getting adequate market share or enough promotional exposure to increase their demand. For purposes of inspiration and future innovation, I have listed 36 of the top plant-based fabrics in part 3. It lists exclusively all healthy, plant-based fabrics for apparel.

The 36 fashion fabrics are an archive of in-depth information about each fabric for resource and reference. An assortment of those listed are currently or moderately extinct, as well as being potent and profound with potential. These fabrics are all significant in opportunity and importance. Several of them need to be produced at a more substantial rate compared to the fabrics already in production, because they are not yet produced in the quantity needed for sustainable, mass-production equilibrium, even as popular as some are. The more variation of fabrics on the market, the more medicinal, healing, healthy fashion occurs.

Healthy Fashion does not stress the idea we wear 100% plant-based fashion overnight. A transition-based path is a more promising route to take for overall wellbeing. Healthy fashion is a natural endeavor that everyone participates in. It's beneficial to really tune into clothing with a realistic intuition behind our garment purchasing. Introducing new or more healthy fashion into one's life involves finances, applicable resources, energy, self-growth, and the acceptable and available moment when a piece of clothing or several pieces are ready to be newly present in one's wardrobe. The fashion cycles of a wardrobe are totally individual based on a person's life experience. It's not completely based on trends, consumerism, or financial standing.

This book naturally engages in a gradual process of potentiating fashion for health, by utilizing seasonal, holistic "style" cycles. Healthy fashion, realistically, is not something that can be achieved overnight. That in itself would be rash, unmindful, and not worth it psychologically speaking. It would become a burden.

Current fashion, as much as it needs to evolve, it is to be currently honored in its own right. It is not about uprooting the entire aspect of fashion already trending with the times, much of it is already healthy fashion. We can find plenty of healthy fashion now and from past generations that is encouraging, inspiring, and adds support to our lives. However, it is about including many more health aspects of fashion into our wardrobes, and making healthy fashion standard.

We can become healthy fashion practitioners through our daily dress. It's a creative opportunity to develop and engage in vibrant, healthy fashion remedies. It's a matter of reflecting on how clothing will affect the body and mind on the basis of plant-tech, ergonomics, the five bodies, the fashion archetypes, and so on. Healthy fashion also contributes to a person's mental and physical health via style, design aesthetics, and its overall spiritually divine presence.

This book was written to envision and embark upon a natural yet futuristic path that is made to inspire, and create anew. Ultimately, *Healthy Fashion* serves to elevate human health. If the planet is diseased we are diseased, and vice versa. It's not only a matter of saving the Earth, it's a matter of eliminating human suffering.

How this book works
There are four parts to *Healthy Fashion*:

• **Part 1: Healthy Fashion for the Mind, Body, and Spirit**
Part 1 introduces fashion in relation to each of the five bodies: the physical, mental, emotional, energetic, and spiritual bodies, and how healthy fashion can support the five bodies with specific fashion modalities, healthy fashion remedies, and healthy fashion practices.

• **Part 2: Unhealthy Fashion**
Part 2 discusses unhealthy fashion; from unhealthy fabrics, to the corruption of fashion. It covers negative fashion practices that are not conducive for the mind, body, and spirit.

• **Part 3: Plant-based Fabrics and Dyes**
Part 3 covers the top plant-based fabrics and plant-based fabric dyes for apparel. This is an important resource for both fashion consumers and industry professionals. The fabrics listed demonstrate the opportunity for more biodiverse, plant fibers to be produced on a global, mass scale. It's aimed to inspire, claiming the potentiality of producing these plant-based fabrics for the present and future time.

• **Part 4: The Plant-based Fashion Guide: A Healthy Wardrobe and a Healthy Fashion Industry**
Part 4 includes how to attain a healthy wardrobe. It gets deep into specific, healthy fashion alternatives and solutions. It covers a substantial fashion-in-transition plan. Clothing care and wardrobe essentials are included. It also includes

the sustainable fashion future for modern, healthy fashion businesses.

Overall, part 1 covers what healthy fashion is, and part 2 goes over what unhealthy fashion is. Part 3 introduces the healthy fabrics and healthy fabric dyes for apparel, and part 4 explains the strategy and solutions to make healthy fashion happen.

Healthy fashion for the five bodies: the physical, mental, emotional, energetic, and spiritual bodies

In chapters 1–4 in part 1 of *Healthy Fashion*, each body is clarified and broken down in the book.

Chapter 1: Healthy fashion for the physical body
Chapter 2: Healthy fashion for the mental body
Chapter 3: Healthy fashion for the emotional and energetic body
Chapter 4: Healthy fashion for the spiritual body

The human body's five aspects—the physical, mental, emotional, energetic, and spiritual bodies—are all taken into account in part 1, as I demonstrate how fashion can therapeutically and medicinally treat each of the five bodies. Fashion, made with each of the five bodies in mind, offers a much more detailed perspective on fashion for total body health. Each body is clarified and broken down in this book, with a detailed overview of the complexities of fashion related to each body.

To what is commonly known as the four bodies: physical, mental, emotional, and energetic, I have added an additional body: the spiritual body. I refer to the four bodies as the "five bodies." It doesn't make sense to combine the energetic body and spiritual body together due to the nature of the book. The energy body refers to frequency and vibration. The spiritual body refers to divine consciousness, soul/spirit growth, and enlightenment.

Fashion and the five bodies all working together as a unified whole, holistically provides integrative, beneficial health effects, strengthening the overall health of humans. Fashion for the five bodies gets to the root, as it targets and relieves the specific ailments within each body. Treating the ailments pertaining to each of the bodies with specific fashion healing modalities is a complex yet effective, synthesized approach to fashion for health.

The human/fashion relationship is specifically affected, too, by the interconnection of the physical, mental, emotional, energetic, and spiritual bodies. For example, the mental body synergistically integrates with our physical body, and so on. When the physical, mental, emotional, spiritual, and energetic bodies work together in fashion, it can help combat disease. There is no need for every healing property to be set in place for a garment to be named medicinal, but several healing components at a time need to coexist and merge for healthy fashion benefits to occur.

Healthy fashion for the five bodies is the foundation with which to heal, recover, and transform, as each body corresponds to specific and unique, healing fashion functions. The physical, mental, emotional, energetic, and spiritual bodies make us multidimensional human beings. I treat the human/fashion connection, and fashion working with the five bodies as a multidimensional fashion practice.

PART 1

HEALTHY FASHION FOR THE MIND, BODY, AND SPIRIT

Chapter 1

Healthy Fashion for the Physical Body

The power of plant-tech fashion

"Plant-tech" is a fashion term I developed. Plant-tech is defined as advanced plant-based fabric and dye technology, and the production of these plant-based fabrics to advance human health for planetary evolution. Plant-tech merges nature with technology. Plant-tech is solely dedicated to the optimal development of fashion products made 100% from plants and minerals.

Wearing plants is a concentrated health practice that leads to the modernization of humanity. The plant-tech solution is founded on the textile development of alternative, choice fabrics produced and used for their health benefits, ergonomic function, superior performance, and long lifespan.

Healthy, plant-tech fashion is the perfect alternative to the world's most toxic synthetic fabrics: polyester, nylon, and acrylic, that are currently dominating the textile and apparel industry. A significant root of the problem in fashion is petroleum-based fabric. Plant-based fabrics perform equivalently to synthetic fabrics and dyes, and are substantially more advanced than them.

The top plant-based fabrics that are currently accessible for the mass market:

- cotton
- hemp
- linen
- ramie
- nettle

- bamboo (natural/lyocell)
- kapok
- abaca
- lyocell

There is an abundance of plant-based fabric alternatives to synthetic fabric available. A few to mention: instead of goose-down feathers and polyester-fill for warmth, kapok, milkweed, and cattails are optimal, thermal, plant-down alternatives for cold-weather temperatures. In place of animal leathers, newer, more advanced leathers are being made from plants, cork, seaweed, and more. Carnauba palm leaf wax and coconut wax are plants that produce natural wax textile finishes, offering a waterproof fabrics alternative.

The special human/plant connection has been forgotten in many cultures today. There's a need to wear plants as they were worn in ancient times. This is majorly based on the deep-rooted commercialization and market boom of synthetic fabrics, ever since the 1930s. However, the profitable outcome and economic value of synthetic fabrics cannot positively override the severity of environmental corruption and human health decline that synthetic fabrics are partly responsible for.

Most plant-based fabrics are niche compared to the amount of synthetic fabrics currently being produced. Cotton is not niche, but it is tainted. Nearly all conventional cotton is genetically modified. There's a bigger picture, a wave of opportunity for biodiverse, non-GMO, plant-based fabric varieties. These various plant-based fabrics cannot be overlooked just because of the current demand for polyester and Bt cotton.

About 80% of all textiles were made of hemp before the 1820s. In the 1820s the cotton gin was invented and cotton fiber took over. Synthetic textile production began in the 1930s and has only increased in production ever since.

In the early 1990s the "green movement" began with themes

of natural fabrics substantially made for the sector of bohemian style market and for bohemian culture. This movement is still current yet niche. It was influenced by the 1960s and 1970s hippy and tribal, relaxed-fit apparel. Bohemian, organic, plant-based fashion is found mostly in natural health markets, New Age shops, or online marketplaces. This green movement, however, is currently less bohemian-dominant, as a new range of plant-based fashion is being produced, catering to many different style genres. Healthy fashion will blossom in a suitable way when it's catered to the numerous fashion styles for individuals' unique needs.

Plant-based fabric diversity

Plant-based fashion fabric varieties should be treated like they are an herbal antidote. For example, people do not typically respond from taking one herb alone. Taking a variety of herbs or herbal combinations, and herbal rotation is typically recommended. It's essential to utilize the plant kingdom entirely for apparel use. Producing textiles predominantly from two plants, like cotton and linen, does not cut it. Many other plants and plant species can contribute to a healthy wardrobe. Cotton and linen are virtuous for their healing properties. They are healthy fabrics, yet there needn't be a reason to dismiss the hundreds of thousands of plants, and the multitude of plant-fiber options that live among us.

The discovery and use of new plants will provide more function and more purpose for apparel. Additionally, using multiple different types of plants, and turning them into fabrics will reinforce economic growth for both developed and underdeveloped countries and regions. Plant-based fabric development over conventional, synthetic fabric development will renew fashion businesses, and it will yield automatic improvements for the industry and other industries. We have to be consistently aligned with this plant-based, "green" movement on a collective scale, and be reassured that plants protect us and support us optimally.

The textile industry, realistically, needs to produce more plant-based fabric types. For example, there's never enough cotton velvet available, and people love their velvet fabrics. We could easily be wearing more cotton velvet, instead of poly or rayon velvet. Additionally, we can discover and develop other plant fibers that can be made into a velvet fabric, apart from the usual cotton velvet.

The need to advance and develop textile machinery in order for new, plant-based fabrics to be industrially manufactured

Before cotton and synthetic fabrics became a popular choice, stem and leaf fiber plants made into fabrics were produced all over the world. Linen fabric is fairly popular and continues to rise. However, fabrics like hemp, ramie, and natural bamboo are paramount textiles for the future of plant-tech fashion. They have less relevance today yet are currently gaining ground and continue to rise.

Based on the textile industry's past and current trends, plant-based textiles (except cotton) and plant-based dyes can give off a misleading, minimizing impression and even appear as exotic, and unattainable to be mass-produced. The current minimal demand for plant-based fabrics makes it clear that they may not appear as important as synthetic fabrics. They are usually recognized as artisan-made and small batch production.

Many artisans from different countries work with many different types of plant fibers other than linen and cotton. That is why it is important to work with the artisans, and expand and develop their textile machinery to produce these multiple types of plants, and turn them into plant-based fabrics. Also, many of the types of plants originate from specific countries.

We have to produce the fabrics where the plants are found. Prizing old-world machinery for the notion that we would lose authenticity and cultural roots keeps us away from modern, plant-tech fashion. Additionally, it keeps countries underdeveloped. Stem and leaf plants aren't contributing enough due to the industry's lack of advanced machinery for their industrial production. So, it's not likely that present-day, traditional textile production, and the methods in producing these various plant-based fabric varieties will prevail. Machinery development and technological improvements for plant textile manufacturing establishes increased textile production with high efficiency.

Rarely are plant-based fabrics and dyes showcased as being produced for the mass market. The ads, especially, give off a limited perspective, limiting any prospect of visualizing the vast plant fiber varieties to be produced on a large scale. There are many misleading impressions of plant-based textile production. For example, dyers and textile producers harvest small amounts of materials from the forest and land.

Requiring the use of small pots over a fire to plant-dye fabric, or weaving on a historical textile machine which takes 10 hours a day to make one yard of cloth, these all minimize the idea of achieving mass quantities of plant-based textile production for the greater good. But in actuality, it can be even more of a reality. It is feasible and it is happening. Currently producing many plant-based fabrics would be labor intensive and off-putting because more necessary, advanced machinery needs to be developed.

Using traditional textile machinery leads to inefficiency and unproductivity. It isn't lifestyle driven. No one should need to be indebted to weaving fabrics on a hand loom, spending innumerable amounts of time producing a yard of fabric. This takes their time away from family, their other lifestyle interests, and other lines of pleasurable work that would ultimately foster a more creatively diverse lifestyle, and this should be available to every person.

If a garment is made as a piece of fine art or as a very exclusive, art-based, collector's clothing item, that's one thing. But the industry needs to consider the artisans and textile manufacturers from all around the world that make fashion products could be dressing 7 billion people in plant-based fashion, if they were equipped with more advanced machinery. When artisans and textile manufacturers are given, or have acquired advanced textile machinery, or have the opportunity to develop these machines, rather than the sewing equipment and textile machines that were made generations ago, strides will be made.

Artisan-made fashion has its place, but look at the dated sewing machine as an example. Before the 1920s and the invention of the electric sewing machine, a treadle was needed to run the machine. It is a bit dangerous to sew with both hands and pedal with two feet simultaneously. Instead of pressing on the footer with one foot, both feet have to move back and forth while the person sews with both hands simultaneously. This takes too much energy, is less efficient, and is a potential danger. The treadle sewing machine is dated, and no longer being used in industrial production, but they are still currently used in many cultures traditionally, around the world.

Eliminating dated textile machinery should be done by almost all major textile and apparel manufacturers. The removal of them should also be accounted for, even by cultures who are preserving heritage with this dated machinery. The sacredness of cloth-making and sewing can still be effective when advanced machinery is used. All cultures have to rise up together.

Petroleum-based, synthetic fabric is not the future

Currently, the fashion industry is the second most polluting industry in the world, the first being the petroleum oil industry. The prime reason fashion is the second most polluting industry is because petroleum oil is used to make synthetic fabric. For this reason, plant-based fashion needs to eventually replace synthetic fashion. It's a matter of medicinal, plant-based fabrics and fashion for health coming into trend. When healthier, modern fashions are put on the map it will go beyond trend or niche. It will be the new fashion standard.

Chemical companies had launched synthetic fabrics and dyes during the industrial boom. Worldwide, the population is persistently inundated with synthetic fabrics in both warm and cold regions because of its cheapness factor, high-speed production turnover, and the economy. They are so readily accessible because they are cheaper to produce and cheaper for the consumer. The cheap product's markup keeps it a highly profitable material.

Too much synthetic textile production has been done creating uber, high-tech plastic fabrics that essentially slow-pollute the body. Because of the variety of modern surface textures and fabric styles the brands and textile manufacturers produce, they are able to promote synthetic apparel as futuristic. Vinyl, latex, and faux fur are examples of fabric types driven to exploit what futuristic style should really be meant for: plant-based fabric varieties. Overall, synthetic fabrics can be made modern in appearance, yet the materials used are not modern.

Petroleum-based fabrics dyed with petrochemicals are made with advanced machinery treated to be continually improved. This machinery and technology need to be put towards the advancement of plant-based fabrics, as they are life-giving. Producing plant-based fabrics instead of manufacturing synthetic fabrics will revamp our ecosystem while reducing chemical factory pollution, smog, chemicals in waterways, and more.

Textile technology prominently contributing to synthetic textiles has created too much synthetic fabric heritage. There are thousands of different synthetic fabric types available on the market. Variations of their style, texture, surface appearance, knit, and weave make it appear like they are different fabrics, but all are of similar or identical chemical composition. There's a definite need for increased plant-based fabric and dye production, and a need for continued advancement of plants for apparel use made in a technologically driven way. As plant-based fashion grows, it will be a major archive of health-supporting fabrics crafted with a multitude of medicinal properties, accessible to all.

100% plant-based fashion: is it feasible?

Yes, it is certainly feasible. Entirely. When we choose to have a plant-based wardrobe, apparel production will decrease, because we will naturally have a smaller selection of plant-based clothing. If we have a comfortable wardrobe made of plant-based fabrics, we won't feel the need to keep purchasing new clothes, and this will decrease fast fashion production.

Plant-based fabrics and animal-based fabrics had dominated the textile market before the 1900s, but their production rapidly declined with the invention of synthetic fabrics like polyester, nylon, and acrylic. Cultivating wild and farmed plant fiber crops gives back to the Earth, and to us, because they are life-giving and highly renewable. Crude oil takes thousands of years to produce, this makes it non-renewable and life-taking. Synthetic textile production is not a sufficiently closed-loop practice. "Plant-tech" fabrics should be the leading dominant material, rather than polyester that pollutes the Earth, and it would cut down on carbon emissions.

A few major ways to boost plant life for textile use are: permaculture, wild plant harvesting, multipurpose plant crop farming, using plant-based food by-products, and aquatic plant farming in the ocean and in other bodies of water. This does not take away from the Earth and its resources. It is an energy exchange between humans and plants. Drilling into the Earth for decayed fossil fuel, and turning it into a fabric does not particularly positively engage in human health. An issue with extracting petroleum oil is that the Earth's body is being drilled into and causing cracks and fissures. On a symbolic scale, this could be considered a wounding of the Earth. Additionally, animals and sea life all suffocate when oil is spilled.

People have reason to believe that lab-grown textiles may help. These materials, as niche products, will reduce synthetic materials but they are not the predominant solution for the textile industry. It is simply not kosher to turn the Earth into a lab. The less artificially made, the better. The production method of growing textiles involves artificial engineering that does not usually yield completely favorable results. More genetic, artificial engineering will ensue. Taking the DNA of a plant or animal, and breeding it is artificial. We have to work with the sun, soil, plants, and plant harvesting in its natural constitution as much as possible. Bio-based fabrics are great, they are still made of plant materials from nature, but lab-grown fabrics are a different story.

It is likely hard to imagine how Earth's own "plant covering" can cover everyone, and there is debate as to whether the planet can hold enough crops for 100% plant-based apparel worldwide. The global human population has grown from 1 billion in 1800 to 7.7 billion in 2019, which could make going 100% plant-based seem like a daunting task.

Some say there is not enough land to produce plant fibers for a 100% plant-based textile and apparel industry. This is not true. There's plenty of unused land to start introducing more linen, hemp, ramie, nettle, and bamboo farms. There's a lot of untapped land on Earth that can be utilized. Desert land can farm cactuses for agave and aloe fabrics along with other desert plants. There are wild forests everywhere. We can make agreements to be gentle with the land, and not strip it bare.

Additionally, much of our land and crops have been destroyed. Plants give oxygen and the planet is in need of that. There is so much land where plants were removed in major urban and suburban areas. We can add more plants elsewhere to compensate for this, and harvest crops, both wild and cultivated to regenerate the environment. The entire process of going plant-based is perfectly natural and healthy for the environment. If you look at jungle plant life, it becomes true that the more plants there are, the merrier, and this a health aspect of the jungle.

Much of the Earth is water-based and is an unused and wasted resource. The ocean is an untapped resource, covering 70% or more of Earth. If we are allowed to share the land with plants and animals, the ocean, lakes, and other bodies of water can be shared too. Seaweed varieties can be developed into fabrics and textiles. Sea vegetation is self-sustaining. Scientists and textile designers have propelled the production of textiles and dyes made from algae and seaweed. Currently, there is a seaweed/beechwood lyocell fabric on the market.

About 70–80% of the oxygen in the atmosphere is produced from all marine plants like seaweed. Harvesting seaweed for textiles will help ocean conservation. Seaweed-based fabric helps the human body to breathe. Furthermore, new developments of hydroponic plant farms and aquatic, wetland plant harvesting also yield a great opportunity for plant-based textile production.

Permaculture farming

Adapting permaculture practice into plant-fiber crop farming will help keep the land wild. Cultivating the area with all the other natural resources co-existing together is a sustainable opportunity. Permaculture-style farms harvesting multiple-use plants will alleviate land consumption. For example, crops like hemp, banana, and coconut are multipurpose plants that can be used for food, apparel, cosmetics, and hygiene products. Practicing permaculture with the land, spreading seeds, and adding plant life to help promote other plant life to prosper can offer more harmony within the plant kingdom. An ethical way of harvesting, for instance, is taking only one or two thirds of the plant so it can continue to sustain itself.

Using natural waste plant resources for our textiles

Natural waste plant resources are to be used for greater gain. Acorns and pine cones have been tested and successfully produced for textile and dye use. They are a by-product of a tree's life-cycle. Acorns are currently being used for textile dyes in large quantities. Pine needles are currently being processed into a viscose fabric. There have also been successful studies of it being used as a new wool alternative. Soil and clay are natural minerals currently in minor production as a textile dye. Crystals can be crushed to extract their pigment for textile dye.

Fabric made from wild weeds

Weeds for textile use are an untapped resource. Wild "weeds," also known as invasive plants like cattails, water hyacinth, flowers, seaweed, stinging nettles, and vines such askudzu, can all be cultivated for more biodiverse, plant-based fabric variation. Based on their rapid regrowth and self-sustaining properties, there's no question this will help continue weed plant fiber cultivation and ensure its permanent reuse. The possibilities are vast.

Plant-based fabric capabilities

Hemp, ramie, nettle, linen, and natural bamboo are a few fabrics that can decrease the demand for synthetic fabric. They will also decrease the demand for genetically modified Bt cotton. We do not have to rely on cotton, but currently we do. At present, cotton cannot cover 7 billion people worldwide. That would be a lot of stress on the plant and it would take its toll on the cotton crop. There's already an unreasonable responsibility put on the cotton crop, and there's an assortment of contributable plant vegetation essential for a modern wardrobe. Cotton is an important fabric, but it's not the only plant among us that can help clothe the masses.

The ideal for fashion is plant-based fabrics made in their most natural state. However, it can be highly valued if the correct measures are used to convert plant fibers through more thorough textile processing, like a lyocell process, as long as the conversion method does not require drastic change of the original material, and it is kept healthy.

The process of producing viscose, a regenerated cellulose fiber, artificially alters the plant ingredient too much. Lyocell is an improved version of viscose, and a healthy one. However, not all lyocell fabrics are created equal. There are certifications that help detect which lyocell fabrics are low-impact, for the health of the body and the environment.

We don't have to focus entirely on plant-based fabrics produced in their most natural state. We can make more use out of the spinneret that's typically used to make polyester. When the melted plastic passes through the spinneret a thread is made. This can be utilized with plant materials. Ideally, we can use other plant materials and types of nature-based ingredients to create more regenerated fabrics similar but different to the lyocell process. Rather than using a chemical solution, however, more nature-based chemicals and non-toxic chemicals need to be developed to make a fabric suitable. This will ensure increased development for healthy regenerated fabrics.

Various methods can be achieved to create modern, healthy textiles. For instance, seaweed would be a health-fortifying textile made in other ways apart from the commonly known, patented Seacell™ fabric. Seacell™ is made of seaweed powder infused into the cellulose-based, wood-pulp fibers. Another innovative fabric could be created, like a fusible web seaweed fabric. This could offer a new way to wear seaweed.

"Plant-tech" fabric health benefits

Plants oxygenate the Earth whether they are on land or in water. They also store oxygen. Humans can't breathe without plants. It would be justifiable to wear plants, as plants give the body increased oxygen. The pH value of plant-based fabric works with the pH value of the body. We are essentially of similar composition to plants. They are the correct extension for the body's "second skin." The body is made of the same elements as the Earth and Universe. When the body is covered with natural resources such as plants, minerals, and water, it can be compared to the way the Earth is covered in plants, minerals, and water.

Natural, plant-based fabrics actively purify and cleanse the skin, supporting the body's natural filtration system. Skin is constantly purifying itself in conjunction with clothing. As the body naturally regulates temperature by sweating, and the sweat releases toxins and acid buildup in the body, the natural fabrics worn help the skin to breathe and allow the sweat to evaporate quickly.

The warmth factor of fabric and the current plant-based thermal fabric selection

No matter the cause, staying warm with synthetic fabric is more important than wearing plant-based fabrics that aren't temperature-sufficient. Reliance on synthetic and wool fabric for their thermal properties will need to persist until the industry begins producing more plant-based apparel for cold weather. As much as plant textiles are celebrated here in this book, and I feel it is a necessary need for health's sake, if temperature-sufficient, plant-based apparel is not available then we must wear synthetic and animal-based apparel for now.

The lack of plant-based apparel for cold temperatures is an issue to consider. Currently, minimal options are available because the demand has not arrived. This leaves people on the hunt for something not entirely available. New textiles need to be developed. Being resourceful, open-minded, and tactful through creative improvisation with our current materials available is necessary for now.

An essential strategy of plant-based, cold weather fabric substitutes is outlined in the plant-based fashion guide. It ensures success for a plant-based fabric future. It is possible to be 100% plant-based, but for the most part, currently, there is a transition period before the industry realistically catches on and manufactures fabrics made from a variety of plants, for all temperatures and for all occasions on the commercial level.

Fashion inspired by ethnobotany and plant medicine

Ethnobotany is the scientific study of cultures and their customs, traditions, and spiritual use of plants. Eastern indigenous, Western folklore, and Native American tribes made plenty of use of plants and herbalism for medicinal purposes. For centuries, plants were considered the paradigmatic form of reason's existence.

The coevolution between humans and plants dates back thousands of years. There's a synergistic relationship between humans and plants, we can't survive without them. We are genetically made to wear plants, and we are naturally drawn to them and nature. There's an interrelation between humans and plants that form a relationship. A natural, healing process occurs through the interconnection and communication we have with them.

Cultures from all over the world use sacred plant medicine for ceremonial healing. Plant medicine is used in shamanic practices. Shamans can interpret a plant's abilities, and they say plants have the power to connect us to the very essence of life. Plants are the gatekeepers to other worlds. Plant spirits are, to some extent, messengers of Great Spirit, and can become a channel used to reach higher realms of existence. Plants used for medicine heal the mind and body on multidimensional levels.

Plants are natural healers inside and out. Studies prove that nature is the most calming and inspiring form of support for mood and emotions. Wearing plants can prompt a therapeutic, human/nature connection. There have been several studies on the beneficial effects of plants and natural scenery placed in hospital rooms. The studies revealed a quicker healing process for the ill patients in recovery.

Plant-based fabrics enhance a human's energy field. They balance the body energetically, on unseen but felt levels. A person's vibrational field merges with plant textiles, creating a type of mutualistic symbiosis. They offer a harmonious state of energetic and vibrational intelligence effects. They have a natural ability to surpass, and even transmute residual, low-vibrational energies due to the plant's naturally high vibration. Each plant presents a unique impression and energetic imprint to help cure particular ailments unique to an individual.

Cultivation of plant-based fabric varieties will help enforce more spiritual, plant consciousness in our fashions. The consciousness of plants initiates self-healing. Spiritual properties inherent within a plant are for medicinal and therapeutic use. Plant medicine found in fashion is balm to the soul, an ultimate cure for disease. It is wholesome, holistic, and the future and technology of our day.

Fashion biomimicry

Fashion biomimicry is the study of nature, and the design and production of materials that are represented in biology. It is inspired by, and emulates the designs found in nature, in order to solve human problems. It establishes healthier, more advanced systems of design, as it enables the mind/body/ spirit to have a closer connection to nature. Albert Einstein once stated: "Look deep into nature, and you will understand everything better."

The composition of the human body biomimicking the composition of plant-based fabric

Essentially, the human body is a living ecosystem, and an extension of nature and the universe in its purest form. We are made up of the same elements as the Earth, atmosphere, and ocean. The human body is predominantly made up of 85% oxygen/hydrogen and 15% carbon. The body's makeup is not similar to the makeup of petroleum-based fabric.

Petroleum oil, the leading ingredient used to make synthetic fabric, is made up of about 82–86% carbon, with 1–2% oxygen. This doesn't include the additional chemical additives found in synthetic fabrics that can be considered acidic and carcinogenic. Synthetic fabrics don't match the elemental makeup of the body harmoniously, making them unable to offer the necessary health benefits.

The human body is primarily made up of water, and 60% of the total body weight is oxygen.

Water is made up of oxygen and hydrogen. Natural fabrics have the ability to absorb water while keeping the body feeling dry. Dry, water-resistant synthetic fabrics naturally suppress oxygen. They do not hold in moisture effectively enough for a healthy condition. Wearing fabrics that align with the body's elemental composition creates a better human/fashion coexistence.

Fashion design inspired by nature

Fashion biomimicking nature is aesthetically pleasing because nature is flawless. At the beach, or when hiking or sunbathing, nature is healing and comfortable. Nature-inspired fashions create a spiritual oasis. Flower anatomy, ocean life, plants, and the honeycomb are examples of nature that can influence and introduce new plant-tech, fabric and design techniques to support the wearer biologically, ergonomically, and spiritually.

The web can be imitated and used in fashion design. When wearing woven and knit fabrics, its structure and its symbolism can establish a web of life connection on subtle and more innate levels. Plants weave the cultural universe, the cosmic web of life.

A biomimetic fashion example: gravity-defying flotation fabrics and apparel

An example of a fashion healing modality that is biomimetic, and not typically referenced as such, is the use of flotation apparel outside of water. The light, airy feel of floating is similar to aquatic sea animals swimming and floating under the sea, or a human floating in water. It literally feels divine to float in water. To make one feel they are floating on the surface of the Earth, this feeling can be imitated when wearing poly, feather, or plant-based down filling material.

Floating in water is a calming, therapeutic activity. There are zero-gravity, flotation therapy clinics using flotation devices to relieve stress, and reduce emotional and physical pain. The use of flotation fabrics can spark inspiration and influence our mood and physical condition.

Flotation-like textiles are not only futuristic and modern, they are therapeutic. Puffer vests, jackets, and coats are flotation apparel examples that achieve the feeling of pure lightness and weightlessness. They give the feeling of floating in air, and they effortlessly lift the physical weight, and even the mental weight of the body. Try on a puffer coat. It doesn't matter if it's filled with feathers, polyester fiberfill or plant-based fiberfill, you will notice this lightness and float-like feel, and your mood will lift.

It will be important to manufacture more plant-based fiberfill for apparel use because of their float-like, therapeutic property. Buoyant plant-based fiberfills like kapok, milkweed, and cattails are materials with natural flotation properties. They feel light, airy, effortless, while alleviating stress and tension. Ultimately, this levitation-like property of plant down creates a harmonic balance within the energy field and physical body.

Four element fashion

Four element fashion is based on the four elements: earth, air, fire, and water. It consists of incorporating qualities of these elements in fashion to support the body. Four element fashion is theoretical in practice and an instrumental force of healing when incorporated into fashion.

It also targets feng shui's effective capacity to bring nature's elements and the human's living ecosystem into balance.

When we establish a connection with the four elements through fashion it becomes a deep-rooted, natural way to align with nature. When earth, air, fire, and water are all integrated together within an outfit, they complement each other, and it can only increase fashion's healing power. When all four elements are synthesized together in a design, they express a form of supernatural communication.

Elemental fashion strengthens a person's connection to Earth and to themselves because it's a symbolic representation of the universe. It's interesting to note that astrological zodiac symbols are connected to the four elements. We may have dominant features of an element we like to express through fashion, and resonate with, due to planetary alignments from the time of our birth, and the planets we like to associate with. The development of four element-inspired fabrics and pre-existing four element fabrics works to incorporate earth, air, fire, and water into the fabric for their healing benefits. One way to incorporate the therapeutic properties of the four elements in fabric is to create a fabric development test. For example, a fabric development test can be applied to depict a fabric's mobility, and motion capacity. Mobility and motion capacity of a fabric can be considered a therapeutic property of the air and water element, as air and water flow.

There are numerous ways to utilize four element fashion. Take the visual senses pertaining to the air element. The air element is incorporated into fashion when editorial fashion shoots capture fabric in motion, or a fashion film interprets clothing in motion with its movement expressed. These both have visual and tactile sensory behaviors of the air element property. Fabric in motion can lift the heart. For example, an extended shawl scarf flowing in the breeze, this can make emotions immediately arise. The movement of cloth is merely one type of expression that we can use to alter health positively.

Four element and feng shui fashion

Four element fashion is largely inspired and influenced by feng shui. Using feng shui in design is a very intuitive, natural way to design apparel. Feng shui, closely linked with Taoism, is an ancient art and science originating from China. Objects, materials, and design elements are positioned to balance and harmonize the energetic forces of the body, the surrounding spaces and the atmosphere. Feng shui uses the wood, fire, earth, air, and metal elements, whereas four element fashion uses the earth, air, fire, and water elements, excluding the wood and metal elements. However, wood and metal are important materials to use in fashion, and are a part of the earth element.

We can apply and incorporate the popular feng shui practice and its philosophy in interior design, and use it in fashion, as clothing is "furnishings" for the body. For example, rearranging the direction of style lines (the seams in a fashion design for their visual aesthetic effect) in a design, to create more ambience and ease. Also, designs can be made feng shui, if the design is non-abrasive with smoother edges, or when seams are placed in a balanced way. A non-feng shui design, for example, is the cut of a garment, and the silhouette's edges and angles obstructing the design.

Feng shui in fashion honors the art of placement in design for balance and energy flow. Space value within design can be a healing property contributing to energetic flow. There's a visual/physical component of space value in design. When design placement is incorrect, this can lead to disharmony.

The four elements strengthen and reinforce inner and outer surrounding energies. Simple adjustments that are made and often overlooked promote ease as well as clear the energy body. Designs can produce flow, circulation, and activate the meridians, also known as the "energy highway" of the body. When a garment is designed without the feng shui principles in mind, it can disrupt the chi energy that flows throughout the body, creating energy blocks.

The yin/yang theory incorporated in fashion design
The yin and yang philosophy of balance in four element fashion acts as an integral part of achieving masculine/feminine balance within a look. Anything designed with extreme polar opposition will not have a balanced, therapeutic effect. Extreme opposition is a form of dualism, and it can disrupt a person's masculine and feminine energies. The hyper-contrast of an outfit being made to look too feminine or too masculine decreases yin/yang balance. A look can be masculine or feminine dominant, but there's a fine line, and sometimes

either masculine or feminine design details can overtake the design. A hyper feminine look and a hyper masculine look is sometimes good, it's just more balance is needed sometimes. The left side of the brain is masculine dominant and the right is feminine dominant. The combination of masculine and feminine design elements merged in dress balances the hemispheres of the brain and the body's yin/yang energies.

The genderless trend neutralizes the yin/yang energies within the body to a certain degree which can cause energy depletion. Genderless fashion can go to extremes and disrupt the yin/yang theory. For the most part, there will be times to celebrate unisex apparel, but "unisex" does not imply "genderless," there is a difference. Unisex clothing is another thing. With the correct intent, unisex clothing, not genderless clothing, could be emphasized as a way to improve gender equality and biased thinking.

Oftentimes, clothing needs both masculine and feminine characteristics and behaviors of style within a look, and this is carried through into unisex clothing. Genderless apparel doesn't meet the standards for the yin/yang aspect of four element fashion. Genderless clothing creates too much blandness, too much obscurity, which results in a look far too outdated, and a type of androgyny that is of limited value.

The four elements introduced in fashion design and apparel

Included below is a sample list of the four elements: earth, air, fire, water, and their properties to be used in fashion design. This is for the purpose of having a better understanding of how the four elements can be fused into a fashion design. A small sample of the colors, fabric types, design details, and therapeutic properties connected to each element is described. This sample list is a small introduction of four element fashion as a healing fashion therapy. Evoking the four elements into a wardrobe or fashion collection creates balance and is a form of elemental alchemy.

The four elements and their properties to be incorporated in our fashions:

EARTH plants, mountains, earthquakes, rocks
Color green, brown, black, earth tones
Fabric type woven, natural, angular, textured
Design detail structured patterns, layers
Therapeutic property grounding, growth, expansion

AIR wind, vortex, tornado, ocean tides, galaxy
Color yellow, gray, blue, white, silver, prism
Fabric type breathable fabrics, mesh, outdoor apparel fabrics
Design detail pleats, vents, buoyant bias cut, fluid patterns, symmetry
Therapeutic property mental release, balance, intelligence, evolution

FIRE blazing sun, fire, heat, energy
Color red, orange, gold, violet, smoky colors
Fabric type thermal fabrics, glossy sheen, flowing fabrics
Design detail vibrant, invigorating patterns
Therapeutic property spiritual cleansing, space clearing, creativity

WATER ocean, rain, waterfalls, movement
Color blue, aquamarine, sea green, black, iridescence
Fabric type stretch-based fabrics, knitwear, athletic apparel
Design detail lucid patterns, soft angles, shimmering fabrics
Therapeutic property emotional release, flow, intuition

Ergonomic fashion

Ergonomic fashion is an innovative design engineering technology. It is the science of advancing product design for its optimal use. So, ergonomic fashion is about creating fashion designs for their efficiency, comfort, and ease. It improves physical, mental, emotional, and spiritual performance. Used daily, it can be a transformative, long-term health solution.

Superior, ergonomic fashion design is sensitive to the treatment of the mind, body and spirit. It's fashion design that adapts to the body and environment for an ultimate mind/body/fashion connection. Ergonomic fashion makes a person feel effortlessly confident. It's a luxurious, comfortable, all-in-one therapy. Life becomes more manageable when our clothing is ergonomic.

Several design details found in knitwear, dancewear, intimate apparel, swimwear, activewear, and outdoor apparel are ergonomic. A lot of it is ergonomic because of the attributes of their technical fabrics. High-tech, ergonomic-influenced activewear is available, but the materials used are typically non-ergonomic synthetic fabrics.

Therapeutic clothing is a clear example of ergonomic apparel. The medical and apparel industries are developing and producing therapeutic apparel such as compression socks for diabetics, seamless clothing for chronic skin conditions, and weighted tops for those with neurological disorders. They can benefit any wearer, whether one has a serious ailment or not. They need to be produced in mainstream fashion, and be worn by the general population.

Non-ergonomic fashion creates a static, rigid, constraining feeling that restricts movement. For example, uncomfortable products like heels, belts, underwire bras, watches, and tight-fitting woven suit jackets are non-ergonomic. However, they can be redesigned into irreplaceable, ergonomic designs.

People can become immune to sacrificing their comfort

for the sake of fashion and style. Examples of non-ergonomic apparel: tight pants with a metal button pushing into the stomach, scratchy zippers that leave marks on the skin, tight belts to cinch in dresses, men's leather belts suppressing breath flow, men's ties pinching at the neck, and woven suiting with no give.

The inconvenience of non-ergonomic fashion is an issue. From embroidery scratching the skin, to tags poking at the neck and hip, and socks so tight that red marks appear, and seams of clothing creating indents, all of these problems may seem minimal yet are disruptive to the day. The mind and body are numb to many fashion irritants. The issues are not always entirely noticeable yet become bothersome throughout the day. Non-ergonomic fashion consciously or unconsciously wastes energy, therefore supports the likelihood of a less productive and less harmonious day.

Ergonomic fashion makes a true statement. No matter what a person's daily physical activity is, whether one is active or sedentary, ergonomic fashion plays an important role. Everyone is active, even when still. The very motion of body cells is constantly moving and performing. Ergonomic fashion works on that level.

Ergonomic fashion eliminates the needless pain, irritation, and negativity of non-ergonomic fashion. It's effortless to wear and perform in. People feel beautifully at ease with themselves when they don't need to fight or struggle with an outfit. Sacrificing style for comfort is unnecessary. In a fashion emergency, yes, and maybe on occasion, but for the most part, daily ergonomic outfits that provide comfort and energize the body are essential.

Ergonomic fashion is about efficiency. The fabrics, apparel designs, and types of garment silhouettes can provide energizing effects, making the day more productive. It can be as simple as wearing a breathable mesh fabric, or a bright colored garment. Everyone wants more energy. Improperly designed clothing can lead to fatigue. There may be a rush of energy like a sugar spike when one is wearing sacrificial, non-ergonomic fashion, but it's an artificial rush; the pain and fatigue settles in soon after. Taking off uncomfortable clothing and putting on ergonomic clothing can provide relief.

Ergonomic fashion is comfortable

Design aesthetics play a role in ergonomic fashion. An aesthetically driven garment with a pleasing appearance becomes a transfer of ease. It harmonizes mood, supports temperament, and strengthens mental health. Modern design doesn't need to compromise comfort for aesthetic appeal. Often, a design's comfort property is sacrificed for its aesthetic appearance. Over time these pieces will be kept in the closet because people want to choose more comfortable, ergonomic pieces.

The style genre, athleisure, is ergonomically designed, and a semi-permanent trend that is influenced by activewear and streetwear. It was brought about because people identify with the need for comfort and movement. Not all athleisure design has high aesthetic appeal because of its simple technical design, but its comfort supersedes its aesthetic appearance. A lot of athleisure design, however, looks modern.

Athleisure is not just a trend; it's a part of fashion's evolution. The world is changing. Designs that constrict the body don't work anymore. Typically, you'll find workers with a formal dress code changing into their sneakers immediately after work, or wearing them during their break-time walk. It's not simply for comfort value; it's functional. Wearing daywear that's a hindrance to a person's daily performance is a distraction and a sacrifice.

One ergonomically designed look that made a huge fashion statement was Coco Chanel's stretch knit suiting. The vintage jersey knit suit was created by Chanel in the 1920s. She liberated fashion. Her designs supported a movement-based, comfortable, luxurious lifestyle. More and more, stretch knit suiting will be available. It is an acceptable, modern, business professional look, rather than the woven, non-stretch suiting that conflicts with natural movement.

It's medically necessary to wear ergonomic design because it has a natural mobility capability. Wearing constricting garments with no give is a form of imprisonment. Back in the 1800s, women wore corsets, petticoats, and dresses that wrapped around the body with all their bulk. The silhouette in that time period was never realistically functional. It had to have been disruptive and exhausting to wear. The puffiness of the dresses kept a person still. They were designed with the intent to modernize apparel, yet civilization and different types of sophisticated apparel have advanced since then.

Design properties that make fabric ergonomic:

There are several physical properties of fashion fabrics. It's most essential to address the physicality of a fabric, in order to improve its ergonomic function and performance.

Stretch fabric: Adding stretch fabric to a design, or cutting fabric on the bias, gives people more mobility. Clothes made with woven fabric can restrict the body if they're not fitted correctly. Even with the correct fit, they may still be too constricting to the body. It is the minor details added together that make a garment more luxuriously ergonomic.

Fabric texture: Healthy surface tactility of fabric is important. The tactile sensation of fabrics interacts with major brain receptors and neural activity found in the skin that covers the whole body. The physicality of specific fabric textures can produce a positive mood and a feeling of pleasantness.

Different textures can promote unique, therapeutic sensations that can be a form of physical therapy.

Architectural 3D fabric: Three-dimensional fabrics are important for the future of fashion. The use of three-dimensional textiles in fashion creates more depth and breathability. A few examples are: 3D knitwear, 3D padded clothing, 3D sacred geometric/origami patterns, fabric embossment, and other weaving techniques to create three-dimensional textiles.

Ventilation: The ventilation property of a fashion design can be a part of a garment's design aesthetic. Breathable insulation and double-lined mesh fabrics made to line a garment will create breathability and ventilation.

Thermoregulating fabric: Cellulose has a porous, hydrophilic nanostructure that absorbs and retains water, thus offering thermoregulation. Plant-based fabrics have both conductivity and moisture evaporation properties. They are naturally moist based on the natural absorption property of cellulose fibers. This moisture is very subtle, however, and it doesn't make you feel wet. Moisture within fabric helps soothe the skin. The moisture barrier of a plant-based fabric naturally coordinates with the water-based human body. It supports body temperature and reduces thermal stress caused by cold and heat.

Moisture wicking fabric: Moisture wicking fabrics have the ability to release sweat from the surface of the skin through their fibers. The sweat is transported to the surface of the fabric and leaves the fabric altogether in a relatively quick manner. Natural fabric absorbs sweat; synthetic fabric traps sweat.

Synthetic garments are generally sweat-inducing. Wearing them while active, for the most part, doesn't allow the skin to breathe properly as it traps the sweat. This debilitates performance. However, being wet temporarily, unless you're in cold temperatures, is not a bad thing. Humans are naturally active and sweat daily. It's a cleansing activity to sweat. Natural fabrics know how to react and behave when wet, and they dry relatively quickly. Linen and lyocell can hold up to 20% moisture without feeling damp. Jersey knit linen, lyocell, and bamboo are a few natural, moisture wicking plant-based fabric alternatives to synthetic-based moisture wicking fabrics.

Textile manufacturers have technologically developed quick-dry and moisture wicking fabric treatments for performance-based fabrics, but they are predominantly made of synthetic fabrics. This moisture wicking technology should be a fundamental pursuit towards plant-based fabric development. There is room for new, improved, modern, technical wicking fabric treatments made with plant-derived ingredients.

Ergonomic fashion trims

Many fashion trims cannot perform ergonomically if they are made with synthetic, artificial materials. Additionally, chemicals, pesticides, and artificial ingredients can create an adverse physical reaction in the body, however subtle or extreme. In many cases, for a garment to be considered medicinal and ergonomic, it needs to be made of plant-based materials in their close to natural form. The whole textile manufacturing process needs to be factored in; from plant fiber crop, to its end use.

Superior, ergonomic design is determined by the use of fashion trims that are gentle to the body. For example, zippers made of precious metals like copper, silver, gold, or plant-based bioplastics versus the typical plastic, aluminum and steel zippers. A biobased nylon material made of castor bean

46

oil has been produced, and is 100% biodegradable. More plant-based fasteners can replace some metal hardware that can be too cool to the touch, or metal zippers that can also be scratchy and abrasive. Depending on where the trims and hardware are placed in the design, this is a determining factor for whether it's ergonomic or not.

The ergonomic surface appearance of fabric for balance and protection

A fabric's surface appearance and texture can work as a protective barrier for the body. Take the paint job of a car as an example. A car's glossy, shiny surface creates a protective barrier for vehicles. Most vehicles have a gloss finish. When a dull, flat, anti-gloss, matte finish of a vehicle is visually observed, what happens to a person's emotion and feeling body is very obvious.

The matte finishing gives off a flat, sandy, rough, non-reflective appearance. This finish can sometimes give a person a feeling of danger because the color is fuzzy, slightly hidden and it's hard to detect the car as it blends into the background. Many types of matte finishes on a car appear to have a depressing, dull look, and stagnant energy to it. People can possibly become discouraged simply from the sight of this dull finish, and it can make a person feel uncomfortable and "off."

The gloss finish of a car, however, is creating a slip-off, protective barrier. This glossy-look makes people naturally feel good, as it's not only visually pleasing, it keeps people safe on the road, as the car paint and finish is easy to see. We can mimic this ergonomic, car paint finish in fabrics. Not everyone is going to wear polished, shiny fabrics, but there's a variety of textures and surface appearances that have protective properties other than glossy fabrics.

Fabric finishing in formal attire, costumes, and dancewear is typically shiny. Shiny, glossy fabrics are used when celebrating a certain occasion. So, this fabric type is connected to healthy emotions and promotes happiness. This is just one example of fashion protecting the emotional body and mental body.

Shiny jewelry and gemstones were often worn to attract the "gods" or supernatural life-forces. Wearing glistening fabrics is not only celebratory; they are working to support the physical, mental, emotional, spiritual, and energetic bodies. A few examples of fabric types that act as a protective layer for the mind, body and spirit: plant-based cotton sateen, cactus-silk, and soft, supple fabrics like bamboo and organic cotton.

Fashion design properties that make a garment design ergonomic:

There are several properties of design that make a fashion design ergonomic. Included below are a few elements of a fashion design that improve its ergonomic function and performance.

Garment silhouette: There are many types of garment silhouettes that support the body, and are comfortable. A few examples of silhouettes that are modern as well as ergonomic; the dolman sleeve, the raglan sleeve, sweatpants, and leggings.

Aerodynamic fashion: Aerodynamic fashion is commonly found in both activewear and daywear. Clothing as a "second skin" is aerodynamic. Ergonomic, fitted base layers form a protective layer, and can be considered aerodynamic, with enhanced function and efficiency.

Compression: There is a difference between healthy compression garments that support the body versus unhealthy compression garments that constrict and suppress the body. For example, some compression garments support organ weakness and help position and hold the organ. They can also help soothe the nervous system. However, some compression garments can restrict oxygen and debilitate the body. This is all up to the design and engineering of the compression garment. Fabric and garment testing is needed to analyze compression garments for their full, health benefit capabilities.

Style line and seam placement: The direction and placement of arrows, lines, patterns, and things that draw attention and energy to north, east, south, west is important. For example, south-directed symbols and design details can be grounding for the observer and wearer. North-directed details offer properties that can connect people to outer space and the universe. Additionally, design details can also produce an energy vortex. Energy vortex-designed apparel can help the chi energies flow through the body. Additionally, symbols and design details can create movement and appear like they are in motion even when they are static.

Ergonomic seamless/seamed apparel: Seamless clothing is popular, especially in knitwear, lingerie, and therapeutic clothing, as they help to heal many debilitating conditions. Seamless knitwear is not labor intensive. They are time-efficient to produce with minimal sewing required, and are very comfortable to wear.

Seams are essential, however. They are decorative and can be used in a design ergonomically. They can be successful in many garments with good pattern-making, while some designs can do without them. Seams can cause uncomfortable friction against skin, creating unwanted sweat, irritation and abrasion. Additionally, having many seam lines in a design causes inflexibility, and hinders freedom of movement. If the body moves freely, more motion is activated and effortless, causing less sluggishness and body deprivation.

There are all kinds of ways to make seams ergonomic.

French seams cover the interlocked threads that can sometimes be a bit scratchy against the skin. Interlock seams minimize rubbing and chafing, and are popular in leggings. Sewing the seams on the outside and using a stretch bias tape to cover them is an interesting technique. Some seam lines could also be specifically placed to offer an acupressure point massage to certain areas of the body. Acupressure clothing performs as a form of acupressure therapy.

Ergonomic fashion for fit and weight fluctuation

Many of the inconsistencies in non-ergonomic design can be addressed by the consumer as they shop for their wardrobe. Incorrect fashions can be resolved simply by shopping for the correct fabrics, and recognizing specific details of garments that comply with a person's individual preference. If something is off about a garment, if it doesn't feel like it's being worn on the body correctly, or if it's not operating therapeutically, it may just be a temporary fix.

For the consumer, it doesn't matter if they purchase high or low fashion, it's the fit that is a major determining factor. Fit can be a challenge, and can lead to a lot of fashion pieces turning over quickly in a wardrobe, turning up in recycling shops, and being thrown away. Fashion that restricts blood circulation and decreases oxygen levels is associated with improperly fitted clothing that restricts movement. That's partly why it's so intolerable to wear clothing too tight.

Wardrobes should include an assortment of ergonomic apparel goods that support weight fluctuation. A person's weight naturally fluctuates by 5–10 pounds or more throughout a given month or months. Males and females will gain weight from water retention and stress. Women during their menstrual cycle will typically gain 3–8 pounds from water retention and hormonal changes. Clothing without enough give bypasses the body's need to naturally fluctuate in weight within a given time. Waste occurs when clothing is thrown out because the body could go anywhere between sizes 0 to 12, fluctuating within months or years. It's not all about one-size-fits-all fashion. It's about creating fashion that's weight-fluctuation sufficient. Transition clothes.

Mental/psychological properties of ergonomic fashion

Mental health can become compromised based on how one tunes into fashion, and how one views fashion mentally in day-to-day life. Fashion is ergonomically balanced and can strengthen mental health when the sensory factors of a design are considered. Materials and their proper placement and alignment create a balanced, harmonious, effortless fashion design.

Improperly placed design details create unnatural or unappealing design. Poor design, in general, can create psychological patterns of control and fear. A lot of styles can be forced, defining who we are with serious misinterpretation. Ergonomic fashion translates part of our personality more effectively than non-ergonomic fashion.

Emotional properties of ergonomic fashion

Emotions are affected by fashion for the wearer and onlooker. The value of fashion used as a creative, natural force to purge, release, and reconnect with our emotions is paramount. Memories and emotions are triggered through the sensorial factors of a fashion's aesthetic. Fashion's deeper motive is to give us access to the recesses of our own mind and present-moment emotions, and allow them to be released or cultivated for health. This makes clothing a channel and an outlet.

Energetic frequency properties of ergonomic fashion

Like music, sound is frequency, just the same as fashion is a frequency one can tune into. The frequency in cloth can be determined by a garment design's silhouette, cut, shape, seam lines, style design elements, and down to the yarn's composition. There are fashions and fabrics out there with an irregular rhythm, creating negative emotions. For example, a garment that does not fit well, it will deplete the energy body, causing depression, anxiety, or unbalanced emotions.

Frequencies found in cloth can alter emotions and mental attitude. They can come in a stripe, the sheen of a cloth; whether it be polished or flat, or a style line shaped in different ways. The continuity, fluctuation, and direction of design elements can also influence a fabric and fashion design's frequency. Measuring frequencies in pattern, print, fabric design, et cetera, can work for the benefit of the wearer. For example, the tightness of a closer-knit weave of a knitted fabric can raise energy and a looser-knit weave can produce calm.

Additional subjects to consider and to be addressed in ergonomic fashion, and how they can be incorporated into dress:

- color
- sound
- lighting
- art
- human/plant connection
- mirrors and crystals

Color: Color is a gateway to mood and emotion. It can evoke and trigger feelings, memories, and behaviors that are subtle or direct. Integrating new colors stabilizes mood. Wearing signature colors is important too.

Sound: Native Americans carried a musical instrument in their pocket and as a clothing accessory attached to their outfit or bag. Whether it was a whistle, flute, or chime, it was sometimes worn to ward off evil spirits. There's a need to delve deeper into therapeutic sound as part of a fashion design, even if the sound is not actually heard.

It's the frequency of sound that matters, like the sound of fabrics rubbing together when a garment is in motion. Fabric, textile dye, the weave of a textile, and embroidery are all critical elements of a design that can create a synergistic effect by their natural or implemented sound frequency vibration. It's similar to a "musical" energy translation and transfer.

An indirect example of sound working therapeutically in fashion is the background music in fashion shows. The selected music can be a serious, spiritual conductor for the clothing collection's theme and mood, and it can be a representation of a person's own style and personality. The musical rhythms of design are a part of the human/fashion coexistence.

Lighting: The sun, moon, and stars represent natural light within darkness. Ocean floors represent the deep, dark abyss of dark colors, while the ocean surface represents the light shining through. We need both light and dark in fashion.

Art: Designers like Coco Chanel, Karl Lagerfeld, and Yves Saint Laurent interpreted famous artworks in their fashion collections. Inspirational art is made to evoke creative expression and spiritual growth. Art creates movement, flow, and an opportunity for change.

Human/plant connection: When you sit in a flower garden it's positive, it's hopeful, there's always happy emotions that arise. When we wear plants, we can attain that human/plant connection and happiness found from a flower garden.

Mirrors and crystals: Mirrors and reflective materials symbolize protection. There is an ancient lineage behind mirrors used to ward off negative energy and be a form of protection. Crystals amplify positive energy while cleansing and purging the body of any residual low vibrations and negative emotions. For example, shimmering mica sand crystals are reflectors. Mica powder is metallic and sparkly.

Fashion and tactile therapy

The development of healthy, tactile-sensitive clothing that supports basic human senses—sight, hearing, smell, and touch—makes fabric and fashion design a therapeutic tool. Tactile therapy in fashion is an important healing fashion modality, because everyone has tactile sensitivity, whether it is mild or severe. Directly and indirectly, we are in constant sensory communication with our clothes. In order to make clothing ergonomic, it should be designed for the body's tactile sensitivity.

There is a relationship between the nervous system and clothing. Sensory nerves are part of the peripheral nervous system. Sensory nerves send information to the central nervous system. The body contains billions of sensory neurons and nerve endings, many of which are directly under and in the surface layer of the skin. The skin's sensory neurons react when cloth is applied, and the nerves are triggered by internal and external environmental changes.

The senses and sensory nerves become depleted and suppressed when we wear fashion that negatively triggers our tactile system (the body's sense of touch). Uncomfortable tactility of fabric goes against the grain of our being. Fabric textures can make us either physically irritated, or physically comfortable.

Depending on the fabric's surface texture, the feel of fabric can transport people into higher or lower states of awareness.

Many textile surfaces induce discomfort. Skin hydration, the body's lipid films, and the skin's surface structure are affected by fabrics that cause stress as they influence active, sensory nerves.

The skin's touch receptors react and respond to cloth, and the following sensations are perceived:

- touch
- pain
- pressure
- proprioception (awareness of the position and movement of the body)
- temperature
- movement

All of these sensations are prompted by the skin receptors. Reactivity between nerves and cloth can trigger a mind/body connection or disconnection. We have to be mindful of our fabric and garment selections, and beware of the sensations that occur from them.

Clothing as a sensory integration therapy

When clothing interacts with sensory nerves, the brain and spine processes sensory integration. Sensory nerves are not always controlled when they are stimulated by apparel. A human's sensory perception reacts negatively to offensive, uncomfortable fabrics, altering mood into unwelcome states of emotion. They send abnormal neural signs to the brain, irritating sensory nerves. This manipulates brain processing and weakens physical, mental, and emotional strength.

We can improve our sensory integration function when we design or wear clothing that doesn't contribute to sensory overload. Scratchy zippers, sticky fabrics, or fabric rubbing loudly are all sensory triggers that disrupt and interfere with a person's sensory processing.

Everyone is consciously or unconsciously managing sensory input, and much of it comes from the fabrics and garments we wear. It doesn't matter whether a person is acutely sensitive or not to specific fabrics and apparel designs, everyone is affected by tactile sensation and the triggers caused by a garment's design. Often, tactile properties of fabric get ignored because of human desensitization and a numbing of the senses. For example, the act of rearranging a garment throughout the day without complete awareness of how it's bothering the mind/body is in part due to human conditioning.

Sound, touch, sight, and smell are a few senses that directly cooperate with clothing:

- **Sound:** the noise fabrics make caused by movement.
- **Touch:** the fabric constantly interacting with the body (pressure, vibration, stretch).
- **Sight:** the visual design aesthetic affecting the body.
- **Smell:** the smell of fabrics, detergents, or chemical treatments in a garment.

Sensory-friendly clothing is unique to an individual. They are also unique to what their needs are at individual moments in time. Sometimes people need the pressure of weighted fabrics, other times people need light, weightless fabrics. Sometimes people enjoy the compression of a tight-fitting tank top and leggings, and other times these people need loose-fitted tee shirts and sweatpants. All different styles of sensory-friendly clothing can be worn and combined together, when needed, for their therapeutic benefits.

There is a need for a sensory analysis of textiles and designs; to test, question, and analyze a fabric and apparel design, in order to be aware of whether it is therapeutic for the senses or not. A design should positively affect a person's sensory processing and help support their sensory input.

There are a variety of tactile sensation experiences, and new ones to be discovered, that can contribute to a multidimensional, and therapeutic, sensory integrative fashion design. This will revamp perceptivity and a healthy interaction between humans and fashion for the mind, body, and spirit. Clothing for sensory integration makes fashion fully equipped, registered as a reservoir of health and healing.

Fashion that supports the body's oxygen levels

People need oxygen to survive. Oxygen-producing, pH-balancing, plant-based fabrics boost the body's blood circulation, stimulate dead skin cell turnover, reduce bacteria and fungus buildup, and support natural breath flow. The skin needs to breathe internally and externally. Oxygen bars and intravenous H_2O_2 (hydrogen peroxide) therapy clinics are beneficial alternative health practices, becoming more and more in trend. Oxygen-producing fabrics can be a part of this trend.

The body is predominantly made up of oxygen. The brain uses 20% of the body's oxygen supply. Lack of oxygen will cause brain degeneration. With lack of oxygen comes disease. Most diseases result in an acidic condition caused by a lack of oxygen. Oxygen deficiency causes hypoxia, low arterial blood oxygen, pulmonary conditions, lung diseases, asthma, pneumonia, hyperventilation, cellular death, and cellular mutation.

Human skin needs to breathe in order to work efficiently. The lungs and nose are not the only oxygen-producing conductors. Skin, the body's largest organ, is a conductor of oxygen flow and oxygen intake. Skin is naturally circulating oxygen constantly. The circulatory system cannot function properly when wearing certain synthetic fabrics, because they create a weakening of the skin organ, causing dysfunction.

Oxygen-promoting fashion is the way to go. The skin needs to be fed with oxygen-promoting, pH-balanced fabrics in order to overcome an unbalanced pH and support organ detoxification. Cellulose-based, plant fibers contain 44.44% oxygen, 6.17% hydrogen, and 49.39% carbon. This combination supports a balanced pH for the body. The skin's acid mantle is slightly acidic in pH, forming a barrier which helps protect skin from bad bacteria and infection. Blood is slightly alkaline.

Synthetic garments add stress to the body, because they trap the body, not allowing it to breathe. However, in very cold temperatures, synthetic garments will not block air flow as much as they will in warmer weather. When oxygen flow is tampered with, the body starts to have an unbalanced pH. The pH level reveals whether a body is acidic or alkaline. When we disrupt the largest organ, the skin, and block it from its breath, it can create an acidic disposition. Additionally, artificial materials are absorbed through skin and can work their way into the bloodstream, causing an unhealthy, acidic pH level.

When synthetic apparel is tight-fitted, it suppresses the body's innate ability to breathe, creating oxygen-deficiency. Synthetic fabric's chemical structure and its fiber formation create a lock, restricting the ability of fabric or skin to breathe. Synthetic plastic fabrics suffocate the body in mild to extreme ways. So, human sweat often becomes trapped between the back of the fabric and the surface of the skin.

Take a plant, for instance. If we cover a plant with plastic cling-wrap, it traps the air. The plant covered in this plastic material wilts and dies within hours if left out in the sun. This same plastic wrap is polyethylene, a material found in synthetic fabrics. The body needs basic nutrition like a plant needs appropriate food, water, oxygen, shelter, and sunlight. Additionally, sea life suffocates when covered in petroleum oil from an oil spill. This is an example of how synthetic fabric doesn't support the body's need to breathe through the skin.

A pulse oximeter measures how much oxygen is present in the body, but we cannot depend entirely on this device to measure levels of oxygen in the body. The body is an intricate, complicated system. There are different levels of defining and measuring oxygen that defy the pulse oximeter. I believe the body is much more susceptible to oxygen deprivation, and can be suffering a lack of oxygen no matter what the pulse oximeter says. Oxygen deprivation may be caused by tight-fitting synthetic fashions, especially.

Water-hydrating fabrics maintain body hydration, keeping the body better oxygenated. Skin is not waterproof. Water-resistant, yes, but not waterproof. When taking a hot or warm shower, our pores open and water is absorbed. Skin regulates water. Keratin, sebum, and fatty lipids in skin help discourage water absorption. Even though the skin's epidermis is naturally water-resistant, skin is still constantly desiring moisture.

Natural, plant-based fabrics absorb sweat, but polyester repels sweat. So, human sweat often becomes trapped between the back of the fabric and the surface of the skin. It has a water-resistant property, as oil doesn't mix with water; it's the petroleum "oil" base that makes it so. The human body is water-based, and synthetic fabrics are oil-based.

Wearing hydrophilic fabrics can support the body's oxygen levels. Synthetic fibers are hydrophobic; they can't absorb water like natural fibers. There is an oxygen atom in every water molecule. It would make sense to wear plant-based fibers that contain water, and are hydrophilic for this reason as it hydrates the skin. Natural, plant fibers are able to keep moisture and water retained in the body away from the skin's surface while keeping the body dry, yet moisturized.

Oxygen is found in every one of our bio-molecules with the exception of carotene and squalene. Within the surface layer of skin, oils, fatty acids and lipids are found. They too contain oxygen. It is also found in collagen and elastin that make up part of the body's tissues. Increasing oxygen to the skin controls free radicals. Studies reveal that cancer can't live in a body that's oxygenated with a balanced pH level.

The body excretes about 1 million dead cells within 24 hours. When we wear synthetic clothing, dead cells tend to trap into the skin more. When dead skin cells are trapped in pores, complications can occur. Skin is a living breathing organ; it needs to be treated that way.

It would be instrumental as well as critical to wear oxygen-promoting fabrics to protect and stimulate the skin surface for better function. Plant fabrics increase circulation and blood flow and improve oxygen deficiency.

Healing fashion

The power of healing clothing is a new wave opportunity and a discovery. Healing fashion consists of curative properties that heal a human's negative ailments. For clothing to be labeled medicinal, healing, and of therapeutic value, many factors need to be considered. Healing fashion conditions the body, neutralizes toxicity, and provides hygiene maintenance. Depending on the health level of fashion used as a treatment, it can help cure the fluctuating conditions of the mind/body/spirit.

The healing activity between injury and cloth dates back to ancient times. Egyptians were not primitive in using cloth to heal injury; it was modern technology. In general, using materials like gauze and plant-based fabrics can be integrated within a design for healing, and help the body recover.

Plant-based fabrics treat and heal wounds. Take an open

wound injury, for instance. Wounds are typically dressed and bound with a natural fiber, like cotton gauze. Healing time progresses when a wound is wrapped in it. Cotton gauze assists in keeping the wound protected, enabling healing and eliminating infection.

The Papyrus Ebers, dating to circa 1500 BC, contains a formula of lint, honey, and animal grease as a topical treatment for wounds. Its absorbent property kept the wound simultaneously moist and dry. Lint is made of very short plant fibers that stick together.

Master herbalists and healers Jethro Kloss and Hanna Kroeger used herbal poultice packs on their clients for the recovery of their internal and external wounds. A poultice is made of cotton flannel and other natural materials as the base. Castor oil, for example, is spread on a linen or cotton cloth and then it's heated. They would also put other oils and herbs on the cloth and place them on the body. The plant-based cloths help release the herbs and oils through the skin's surface, allowing them to be absorbed into the system.

There's a need to place plant-based fabrics on the body for healing and recovery. The cloth is the catalyst and conductor of the poultice treatment. Poultices and compresses speed up blood flow, circulation and yield curative properties. When popular, they were a prime health treatment.

The body is naturally dressed and bound with fabric as a covering. This works to improve circulation, and support internal/external wound management. When we adapt these types of dressings to clothing, better circulation, more lung capacity, agility, balance, and temperature regulation will result.

Cleansing fabric

Natural, plant fibers have a nap that brushes off dead skin cells, rejuvenating the skin. Even at the finest thread count, they still act as a natural skin buffer, creating room for new skin cells to grow. Based on a cellulose fiber's structure, its texture and material is non-abrasive and gentle.

Face and body cleansing cloths made with plant-based materials like cotton, bamboo and coconut are popular. They are made into a plant- and pulp-based, non-woven web and gauze-like fabric. They are not typically made with animal or synthetic fabric. Face and body exfoliators made with plastic, or animal hair, don't seem as hygienic or comfortable.

Cosmetotextiles

Cosmetic fabrics, also known as cosmetotextiles, are fabrics infused with skincare and health care ingredients. They are essentially a great idea. Cosmetotextiles are topical treatments for the body, and it is a technology merging cosmetic formulas and textiles together. Several cosmetic fabrics, and their fabric treatments, support circulation, decrease cellulite, and have moisturizing effects.

The cosmetic ingredients are microencapsulated; they are dipped into the fiber, and are then fully embedded into the fiber. They are released when the body is in action, or the skin and fabric are rubbing together. Companies are microencapsulating healthy soothing and medicinal ingredients such as aloe, jojoba oil, caffeine, retinol, and vitamin E into their fabrics.

There are several companies producing cosmetic apparel, yet there are things to consider because some of them include false advertising gimmicks, and the product might not be as useful as it should be. For example, on the market there are some brands producing aloe-infused spa moisture gloves that therapeutically moisturize the hands. Many of them, however, cannot be a healthy cosmetic apparel item, because it's made with a petroleum-based fabric, and/or its cosmetic fabric treatment is made with harsh and skin-irritating artificial fragrances and chemicals.

Full authenticity and transparency of a cosmetic garment's properties is essential. Some microencapsulations may be artificial or semi-synthetic; the material of the capsules that administer the cosmetic ingredients has to be healthy for the body. They need to be plastic-free because this can cause a problem for the skin.

The natural health food industry trends and their relation to the fashion industry trends

To elaborate on the effectiveness of fashion for health, I relate it to the current trends of the natural health food industry that's creating a healthier constitution for the body. The health food industry is a good source of reference that resembles and parallels healthy fashion. Whether it be healthy or unhealthy, what's being delivered through any business is a reflection of what needs to change on the collective level. Like a natural health food store that serves healthy, natural food with ethical standards, versus a drug store that sells a lot of junk food and cheap, artificial products, it's what a person is drawn to that determines their health.

The health food industry is prospering, moving at high speed with major retailers giving people access to healthy, nutritious foods that combat disease. For example, the USA's west coast shops like Whole Foods, Sprouts and other multi-chain natural food grocers are making health foods widely acceptable and available, and they are on the rise. Fashion businesses, on the other hand, are only in the minor to moderate stages of gaining traction within the community to deliver a fresh, healthy approach that operates like the new, big health food trends. Making healthy fashion more ingrained into the mainstream, and less segregated within the fashion industry, is crucial.

Health food stores are the gems of all grocers. They carry whole foods. Their beauty, hygiene, and herbal supplements are plant and mineral derived. They promote and sell plant-derived fashions. More plant-based fashion brands and fashion business retailers will soon be setting the trend like these mass-scale natural food stores that are providing healthy food options. Additionally, the boosted developments of alternative health sectors in major department stores are on the rise.

The beauty, hygiene, and health food industries are all pretty current, and are incorporating more and more natural ingredients in their products for health and wellbeing. Fashion apparel and fashion accessory trends need to work more along the lines of the health trends of the natural food and beauty industries.

Plant-based fashion is the closest, external, topical application for the body. Like the way food gives us nutrients when taken internally, our fashions can give us nutrients externally. With that said, to flourish internally and externally we can choose healthy fashion as a prominent force to heal the human body.

There are similarities between natural health foods and healthy fashion. Like the food we eat, fashion feeds the body too. The holistic healthcare industry prescribes plants as medicine, and the same should go for fashion. What we put on our body should be as important as what we put in our body. Wearing natural fashion, like eating natural foods, supports health.

Plant-based fabrics are like a health food to feed the body topically. It is likely we are nutrient-deficient, topically, because plastic fabrics are like junk food for our bodies. The textile industry is producing fast fabrics that people are not feeling satisfied with and it is just a quick fix.

Junk food never seems filling, only momentarily. Like denatured foods, synthetic fabrics are denatured too.

The risks of increased ailments, debilitating conditions and disease for a human are decreased through special nutritional diets and herbal supplementation. Hanna Kroeger, herbalist and healer, named the "medicine woman" and the "grandmother of health," she left a wealth of immeasurable wisdom and knowledge through her books and life work. She helped thousands of people through herbs and natural health products. With that said, the focus of natural health and wellbeing, and several other holistic lifestyle factors need to be considered in order to achieve overall health, like meditation, water therapy, hygiene, physical therapy, fresh air, and of course, multidimensional healthy fashion.

Acidic food/Acidic fashion

The power of eating oxygen-rich plants brings the body back to a healthy, balanced pH level. Wearing pH-balanced and pH balance-forming plant-based fabric helps diminish an acidic pH that's responsible for immune system decline. Plant-based fabrics are a natural catalyst to promote a pH-balanced body. The rise of bacterial infections, hormonal imbalance, and a poor immune system is actualized by the use of synthetic fabrics.

Acidic foods are disease-forming. Clothing worn topically shouldn't be acid-producing. A main cause of this acid formation is the 85% or more of carbon content in synthetic fabrics. Synthetic fabrics are not usually oxygen-promoting.

Plant-based fabrics that are pH balance-forming are superior, with textile performance properties essential for health. Studies reveal ingredients like castor oil used as a moisturizer alleviates skin conditions while improving skin cells drastically. Neither does it disrupt the skin's acid mantle. Moisturizers made with castor oil, aloe vera, clay, and salt, cleanse and renew skin. These cosmetic ingredients will also benefit the wearer when added to fabric-finishing treatments and added to laundering detergents.

GMOs in food and fashion

GMOs do not only exist in food; they are in the fabrics we wear. Cotton, soy, and Ingeo™ (dextrose sugar from corn) fabrics are predominantly grown genetically modified. Monsanto, recently acquired by Bayer, was one of the founders that introduced genes into plants, and was a leading, top chemical company in the world. They were a top producer of synthetic textiles, and were one of the initial creators ever since the 1930s. They were also the initial producers of genetically modified, Bt cotton since the 1990s.

Both our food and fashion are corrupted. We need to take back our food and fashion. The progression of fast junk foods and genetically modified foods, including fast junk fabrics and genetically modified fabrics, has taken a tremendous toll on humans and the environment. Consumers are seeking healthier options, becoming more acutely aware of the need to eliminate chemicals in food, and eat more organic foods without artificial ingredients. We need less toxic chemical usage, more low-impact fabrics and dyes, and more plant-based, healthy, non-GMO textiles.

In the USA, the Food and Drug Administration (FDA) requires nutrition labels on most foods. People are taking more notice of what's being put in food. If the textile industry had to create a label with a list of contents a fabric is made of, the product would be more challenging to sell. Brands and consumers may not even be able to identify if the fabric they are purchasing is genetically modified fabric or not, if it's not stated anywhere on the garment. Neither can fashion companies find out what a fabric is made of if it's not listed by the textile supplier.

Vegan fabrics or plant-based fabrics?

"Vegan" is a common term in fashion, supporting animal-free products. However, the term doesn't completely resonate with fashion that is "plant-tech." Vegan fashion is a term used in a lot of greenwashing practice because it currently demonstrates a drive to purchase synthetic products. It can be considered a greenwash practice to promote plastic fabrics as a healthy "vegan" option, because, although it may be healthy to not wear animal materials, it's not a healthier swap to wear plastic. A vegan diet is typically esteemed for its living, plant-based nutrition. So, wearing toxic, artificial fabrics is not completely in alignment with a vegan lifestyle. Vegan fashion needs to be true to its word: plant-based. "Plant-based" is a better term to use over "vegan" due to misconstrued greenwashing of the term. Plant-derived foods contain a living essence. Vegan fabrics made from synthetic, artificial materials don't carry that enhanced, living essence.

Natural plant-dye color variation: in foods and textile dyes

The textile industry mass-produces dyes like the food industry mass-produces processed foods. Synthetic foods are altered with preservatives, artificial coloring agents, food stabilizers, as well as filler items and artificial flavoring used partially for consistency. Some of these synthetic add-ons are included to deliver food with the exact same taste and appearance. The organic, holistic food industry bypasses chemical and artificial processes, keeping foods pure in their original form. For example, some coconut water brands will state on their food label: "Color and taste may vary because of its natural state."

The individual coloration of organic fruits and vegetables, along with their distinct taste, can be marked as a valuable quality. Additionally, no meal, if done creatively, is ever alike. Even when a recipe is followed multiple times, the meal will always taste special, unique and different from the rest of the times the recipe was made. Food doesn't always taste the same; the experience changes constantly.

Conventional, mass-produced textile dyes make unnatural, synthetic colors to such extreme exactness. However, plant-based dyes can be equivalent in their color consistency compared with the consistency of synthetic dyes. There are currently a few mass-scale manufacturers that produce plant-based dyes with color exactness, because they made technological developments in plant dye-extraction methods and machinery.

When it comes to certain plant-based dyes, it might look like natural color variation is too organic in appearance, yet this is something to be celebrated. We can make it appear futuristic and modern by the garment's design aesthetic, and via the correct way of marketing plant-based dyed fabrics. If we can make it look modern, and not all "earthy," it will cater to and appease all consumers. Not everyone wears the "earthy" look. This is where the design and marketing of the product steps in.

Overall, there will be a broader invitation to accept color variation as time goes on. Color variation from plant-based dyeing is a mark of quality and luxury. Color uniqueness can be treated as a special attribute of the garment, and perceived as a limited-edition, one-of-a-kind product that is unique for the individual.

Plant fabrics are more of a priority than plant dyes, at this time. Once plant-based fabric varieties are in place and become a trend and standard, plant dyes will naturally be catching on.

Plant fabrics are a priority that can be achieved at a quick rate. I go into greater detail about this in the plant-based fashion guide, but a great place to start is using low-impact dyes. Chemical dyes can still be used but they would need to be low-impact and healthy. We just need to choose the correct chemicals that are non-toxic. A lot of chemical dyes use ingredients sourced from nature that do not harm or threaten. Merging plants with chemical mixtures, and plant-based chemical mixtures that are not alchemically going to reject or conflict with each other or cause harm to the body, is essential.

Agricultural biodiversity in the food industry

We don't just eat one type of vegetable or fruit; neither do we simply wear one color. Being able to wear different types of plants and have these fabric options is necessary for their differing nutritional, medicinal, and energetic properties. Natural, plant-based fabric varieties are simply not available to the masses, and only a select few are in mass production. It's ideal to have more fabric options to choose from that are made from a variety of different plants.

Thousands of plant-based fabrics made from different plants aren't available, only thousands of synthetic, oil-based fabrics. Eating variation is celebrated across the world with hundreds to thousands of different types of foods and meals to choose from. Through biodiverse fashion we are much more able to have a more well-rounded fashion "palette."

Chapter 2

Healthy Fashion for the Mental Body

Universal fashion

Embracing the opportunity for healing fashion to manifest as a universal initiative will be most beneficial for the collective human consciousness, and will support the mental body. No matter how underprivileged or privileged a person is, not one has escaped the reality of the mistreatments of unhealthy fashion. Second-world and third-world countries take a hit, and so do first-world countries. The fashion industry, driven to create a level-grounded, equal, global population as a whole, will rebuild the new golden age of fashion.

We are all out of symmetry, and it can be observed through what we wear. We are all out of sync together in the name of fashion. As an example, in underdeveloped countries, cultures who wear traditional dress may be producing outdated thinking, and their fashion needs to be updated for the most part. For the more technologically developed regions of the world, they wear modern fashions, but much of it is sacrificial fashion, and this is a popular crime against the body and mind. There's a necessary need for symmetry and balance, and it occurs in universal fashion.

Universal fashion is not cultural appropriation

Cultural appropriation is a culture that adopts the customs, practices, and ideas taken from another culture, and they are used for purposes not intended by the original culture. Many fashion designers are just simply inspired by other cultures, and are influenced by them. The concept of cultural appropriation in fashion is creating a negative boundary. It pushes people away from being able to dress freely. It's a block. Cultural appropriation is an excuse that misrepresents culture and identity.

Not sharing cultural identity creates more segregation. If we can't wear what people from other countries are wearing, it gives people an opportunity to segregate through dress. Traditional clothing worn only within specific countries can cause segregation. It's exploitative to fragment fashion in terms of clothing customs. Traditional dress will always be a part of life. With that, there's an empowering, new movement of embracing universal modes of expressing style.

Universal fashion takes advantage of the many styles from different regions of the world, and their many different types of attire, and merges them together. It bypasses the cultural norms of segregated dress, creating non-segregation. Traditional use of clothing—modernized, and worn by all ethnicities combined—is a part of the universal fashion solution. It's also about purposely bringing different cultural fashion concepts together in union.

It's not cultural appropriation to honor and wear another culture's style. There's no such thing as food appropriation. World cuisine clues people in to the idea that if we eat different foods from other cultures, it doesn't mean we are mocking or imitating their culture; food is universal. Everyone eats Chinese food, Indian food, Mediterranean food, Mexican food, and so on. The value of eating different ethnic foods, and integrating them within all countries, is a part of a universal communion. This concept can also be delivered through fashion with respect to universal fashion.

Advanced, universal fashion is new and fresh fashion designs made to inspire. Clothing will always reflect the history of fashion. Making use of past fashion is important, yet as time naturally embraces modern society, new developments of conscious fashion need to be explored. This will take fashion into a place where all cultures are invited to participate in universal dress.

There will always be elements of traditional dress and costume in fashion, but consciousness moves and so does fashion. If a specific region's fashion and style has been worn as ritual attire for ages, and if it has not been brought into trend and modernized, it is static and at a loss. It can cause a dated, stagnant feeling that interferes with the rhythms of life.

Traditional dress can represent museum-like qualities that attest against trend value, yet societal regimes cause traditional dress to become truly old-world thinking. Every culture, every country's demand on fashion, and any biased thinking cannot remain, as we have to push fashion as universal in order for global balance to occur. It's about embracing universal fashion on the global front. There is a fine line but a strong one for modern fashion to become universally merged in all different cultures, for balance.

Healthy fashion, facilitated as universal, will set the standard for the fashion industry itself within all countries. This will eliminate segregation, racism, discrimination, and so on. There is a need to work together communally in the name of fashion. It is a kind of fashion communion that bypasses segregation. Global balance is about sharing each other's lifestyle to some degree. It is a form of empowerment.

Modern brands that embrace universal modes of expression push boundaries in fashion worldwide. Universal fashion lessens conscious or unconscious judgement and even personal criticisms placed on the different types of fashion; on the styles we wear and the styles of people from around the world. Non-universal fashion alienates people, environments, and societal cultures.

After the time when America was wearing purely Native American fashions, America's traditional way of dress began to be European-influenced, and fashions were exported from Europe. European women wore long puffed-out dresses, petticoats, and corsets. For men, they wore a suit, coat, vest, and hat. Some of American fashion, as it has been for many decades, has become a melting pot possessing universal fashion appeal. The framework has been built of different ethnicities and a variety of ethnic fashion styles that interrelate.

Fashion is like the daily newspaper, exposing where we are at collectively. Cultures need change. This can be done by changing traditional forms of dress, creating a modernist approach to standard, traditional fashion. This establishes modernity as a mechanism to bring diverse cultures together into a state of balance. The pulse of fashion is traditionally non-traditional. Fashion styles stem from tradition yet move beyond tradition into making them something unknown, new and modern.

Social ethics in fashion for global balance

Equality is one of the core values of universal fashion. Social justice creates world equilibrium.

Fashion's socioeconomic impact on a collective scale is a way to solve inequality. It's imperative that a diagnosis and solution should come about for socioeconomic balance, and social health balance. There are hierarchical social dynamics within fashion that resist equality.

There are positions of power in the fashion industry that dominate, direct, and enforce. The two positions of class— high and low—creates a gap, forming segregation. Because of this, several lower-end positioned employees have little to no voice. A major concern is the unethical mistreatment of laborers and workers, working in many different job roles in the textile and apparel industry. Everyone involved in the supply chain is being affected, in both underdeveloped and developed countries all over the world.

Due to unregulated laws, workers may be forced to perform no matter the wage, hours worked, or working conditions.

Some of these workers are typically from a lower class or at poverty level. Some companies from developed countries are utilizing resources from the workers of underdeveloped countries to gain benefit, while suppressing the needs, rights, and welfare of people from these underdeveloped countries. Life expectancy and health vary greatly within different countries. Unequal lifestyles are concerning. The technological development of international supply chains can alleviate the lack of support people in lower-end positions of employment are given.

People who are not getting a fair deal on this earth should be protected. If people are not comfortable financially, they are not receiving a fair deal. For total global empowerment, developed countries cannot use underdeveloped countries and their manufacturers for gain, when their laborers can't even make a living wage. Additionally, fair trade and new forms of money exchange will repair the faulty system that is based on greed, profit, and false power. It's not always about currency; it's also about an energy exchange.

What will be done is the industrialization of underdeveloped countries so they too can develop modernization of society. Companies that are not bogged down by old-world regimes of class and traditional, dated practices, through their technological fashion industry developments, this will ensure planetary evolution. Evolution of society needs to include all communities and countries. The suicide epidemic in India and child labor scandals in China and in other countries are a couple of situations that show improvements need to be made within the industry in order to take better care of the livelihood of people.

People need to be paid sufficiently, have a suitable work environment, to be treated properly, and receive a fair work schedule. On top of that, people should be given additional, supportive rewards and opportunities to develop and grow their future career. People should have options in terms of work and career throughout a given lifetime. Many organizations and programs across the globe are giving workers access to educational programs to help them achieve empowerment. Being a socially responsible company requires specific methods of production, like giving accessible room for every employee to grow and feel empowered. Educational programs, events, campaigns, organizations, and workshops that promote the welfare of those working in underdeveloped countries and impoverished communities worldwide are essential. Naturally, this will introduce more technology and development within a community conducive to a better lifestyle.

Healthy labor practice standards like providing a living wage and suitable work conditions will lessen the control of dominating, cheap, fashion surplus production. Ethics of a humane lifestyle merge with ethics of an appropriate fashion production cycle. So, the ethical consumer can decide to gravitate towards companies facilitating a humane mission.

Ethical businesses and organizations are creating more opportunities and positive initiatives for artisan-based companies and for people living in underdeveloped countries. Building and developing better foundations for businesses in underdeveloped areas ensures better health and more equal opportunities. A society that does not have appropriate food, water, and shelter for all is under dire conditions of the very worst. The fashion industry must be a part of improving everyone's welfare. Tradition is important and may succeed more than modernization in different ways, yet social health proves to be a priority.

Shopping at thrift stores is a protest against retailers lacking social responsibility within their supply chain. The loss of a company's sales will oblige them to address the reason and thus will influence their business practice. It's always fun to sift through racks and find treasurable, unique pieces.

Shopping at thrift stores supports healthy fashion. Purchasing fashions from ready-to-wear designers and luxury brands that maintain small-scale production to achieve the ultimate craftsmanship and quality will help too. Yet, we can wear a favorite tee shirt that took very little time to make and it's just as important and equivalent to a designer item.

Social health will improve when we bring the world together. There's a dualistic nature between Western technology and Eastern philosophy. Slowly, Western civilization is becoming aware of the need for more spiritual awareness often found in countries with strong traditions and customs from Eastern civilization. Eastern civilization is becoming more and more interested in advancing technology like the Western civilization is focused on, and that's important too.

America truly is a melting pot, holding retreats and building organizations of every religion and culture in every state. Christianity, Hinduism, Buddhism, Taoism are a few world religions that are all spread out and accessible to the public in the USA. This can represent the interest and need for cultural integration.

Fashion for global economic balance: artisan-made fashion on a mass scale

Artisan fashion is sacred; there's an art to it. It is realized as a spiritually influenced, health-conscious way of producing fashion. Many artisan-made garments are holistic. They practice traditional methods and make products typically made with genuine materials. Artisan craft is healthy because of the time, energy, and intention put on their products.

Many of these artisans work with multiple types of plant fibers other than linen and cotton. That is why it is important to work with them, and help the artisans expand and develop their textile machinery to produce these multiple types of plants into fibers. Additionally, many of the different types of plants originate from specific countries. In order to produce many different plants into fabrics, we have to work globally.

Small-batch, artisanal fashion production cannot clothe the world population. There's a place for artisanal fashion, but most artisan fashion companies are run on a small-batched basis. There's much more to be done for healthy fashion to succeed in the mass commercial market. When practices of artisan-made fashion are kept, while their traditional methods are updated, making them more advanced for mass production, this will make it happen.

Technological developments for healthy textile and apparel production have not yet reached an absolute. There's not enough technology being implemented or products available for the consumer. Rebuilding and launching these smaller, artisan-based manufacturers into larger-run, manufacturing companies better establishes and grounds healthy fashion socioeconomically for the future.

We have to take full advantage of all that nature can offer. We can make the demand for plant-based fashion by asking for it. When each country contributes, it will happen. When artisan companies and textile companies from each country expand because of new developments in textile machinery that are specifically made to propel biodiverse, plant-based fabric variations, this can become a positive, successful, economic outcome for so many. It is already beginning.

The fashion politics of social classes

Fashion is very much political. Fashion as a political scheme diverts people away from the deeper truths of fashion. Healthy, universal fashion can work as a coping mechanism for people that feel negatively affected by societal regimes that they cannot relate to.

Political schemes are expressed in fashion weeks and fashion shows worldwide. Political forces of fashion announce what's available, determining who gets to wear what by the price tag and its association with a particular social class. This is not to dismiss designer, high fashion or say it's disrupting global equilibrium to an excessive extent. High fashion is made for influence, inspiration, and cultural integration, and there lies its importance. Traditions of fine dress surpass social hierarchical classes, because we can take away the social classes and appreciate fashion as fashion. Yet there really is a need for designer fashion brands to adapt and brand themselves in order to make their clothing accessible to all. Universal fashion celebrates equality.

Additionally, it is politically incorrect to cut costs in production areas where underprivileged employees get the raw end of the deal. There's no fairness when the entire supply chain is not being fair. This is a significant reason why too many underdeveloped countries are not developing at a rate needed for social balance.

Several political, hierarchical regimes are structured to impart imbalance within the fashion industry. Forces of false power within the fashion government support the "hive mind" matrix. This is a system set up to accept hierarchy and the high-fashion class. They amount to a small percentage of the population, and purchase haute couture or ready-to-wear garments for thousands of dollars. Wealth may contribute to the "fashion hype" way of dressing that is built not on personal style but on social status. This creates a false, artificial communication behind dress.

The lower class may be inclined to have a stronger connection with clothing because there's sentiment behind clothes that don't get rotated out of their wardrobe too much, versus clothing that gets disposed of or forgotten in the closet after a few times of wear. The budget-conscious may make do and wear secondhand garments or gently-used clothing, and often they do not complain about this because they establish a special awareness and appreciation towards their clothing and wardrobe. There are contributing factors that could lead us to believe that the wealthy have less of a connection with fashion, in certain cases. Garment disposability is associated with a larger budget.

Is it better to have a big wardrobe, or a minimal wardrobe that includes a selective collection of pieces? For one's mental health, choosing a smaller wardrobe can create a stronger connection with clothing. There's a lot of different wardrobe styles that people have, but choosing a smaller wardrobe is one effective way to break away from clothing hoarding and the human/fashion disconnection that may occur when we have a large wardrobe.

Merging cultures: thinking outside the fashion capitals

There's a large fashion network found in cities. There are thousands of fashion designers and fashion businesses within these fashion capitals. The fashion capitals—New York, Milan, Paris, London, and Tokyo—are fashion-focused, based on their high-density populations and urban cultures. With the rise of industrialization, and with these large city channels distributing fashion, it's no wonder urban fashion is fast-paced, and becoming more so with new technology. Fashion business will always be at the center of fashion capitals, or any location offering fashion shows and weeks. However, fashion businesses create subcultures from other cultures in areas other than the fashion capitals.

Many fashion ideas do not start in the city, they are created from subcultures. Furthermore, there's growth value when fashion is spread throughout countries and regions of all sizes, not merely found in crowded city populations. Societies living in cities that don't always take advantage of what goes on outside of the city is a part of the imbalance in fashion.

Cultural integration is important. Smaller towns and their cultures should be observed and viewed as being a notable contribution and an important part of the fashion scene. Bringing this understanding to the public at large through fashion marketing and advertising is paramount.

The Dalai Lama once said: "New Yorkers, why don't you spread out? You're so congested. There's a lot of land not being used in America." He has a point. This inner-city congestion needs to be channeled in healthier, more balanced ways. Congested populations bring about a specific culture, but one that may not be entirely sustainable for fashion. There is an opportunity to merge urban fashion and rural fashion parts for global balance.

Cities are efficient. There's immediate access to educational resources within a block's distance. Cities are great, they prove to be able to harbor a lot of inspiration through their museums, theaters, art, music, history, literature, but the grandeur involved leaves smaller cities and towns feeling less up-to-date, less able to contribute to the larger cultures collectively. But this isn't really the case. Yet most smaller towns and rural areas aren't fundamentally equipped to offer what city life offers. More balance occurs when there are city-made opportunities in smaller cities and towns. This can come to fruition when they incorporate more modern, healthy, universal fashion.

Healthy fashion consciousness will make all of civilization more balanced. When subcultures within cultures are observed, and fashion businesses are using them to influence their work, and draw inspiration from them, fashion will become much more interesting.

Local community growth on a more substantial basis in rural or suburban parts of the world is essential for fashion evolution to occur on all global fronts. Incorporating fashion trade and resources in smaller regions that are similarly found in large city marketplaces will enforce fashion as a modern form of language-based "currency" or "energy." It is a solid mark of wide-ranging fashion communication for everyone.

The charm of a town ends when their local people's fashion appearance is negatively affected by being on the outskirts of a city, for the most part. Many areas are inhabited by populations that dress in a lower vibration of style. This isn't a description of every town's fashion collectively, or everyone's style and fashion presence individually. In fact, many people within smaller towns wear advanced fashion and incorporate advanced fashion concepts in their looks.

Some parts of cities have a defective negativity, and a greed-based profit accumulation that promotes a corrupt corporate agenda to some extent. There is also health within cities; however, they contain a lot of heaviness that needs to be uprooted through the merging of smaller towns and larger city cultures. This is a healthy, "universal" fashion strategy.

No matter what, on a mass collective, majority scale, everyone has to rise up together. Big city people can learn from small city people, and vice versa. City cultures can be influenced and inspired by town cultures, and vice versa. This will dismantle the dynamics of fashion hierarchy. It's not about which city or town is better dressed; it's about how people's way of dress is being used to alter their life and respective culture.

Social regimes of dress: the uniform

Uniforms, in some cases, can be associated with negatively. Some uniforms can symbolize stagnation, rules, suppression, the outlawing of nature, the outlawing of creativity, and dated traditions. The use of uniforms has spread its roots of defined establishment and social authoritarian status. There is a difference between a uniform that is a specific, special garment that is worn often, that symbolizes a connection to the wearer, and adorns and enhances personality, versus the traditional uniform that segregates, creating an outdated form of judgement and hierarchical status.

Traditional custom costumes around the world are a type of uniform that is being worn as current fashion. They can represent a dated past, that does not support change. This is where, globally, the technologies used in the modern fashion world need to influence and embrace communities that do not represent the fashion times. There's no justice coming from the pains of dated fashion, or sacrificial fashion. Traditional costumes that are held on to too strongly go against the fashion industry made of persistent change. It creates a conflict, and it's a conflict made of resistance. This has become a situation that goes against fashion's holistic cycles.

Variation is important. For example, if the whole world dressed like a monk, in an orange robe every day, the world would be in trouble. A uniform worn in this context is purposeful, and there can be spiritual sentiment behind it, but it's not for everyone. Variation is fun. It breathes life; spreading creativity and cheer.

Uniforms are being worn all over the world. Many of these uniforms are not contributing to insightful design. A fashion design that reveals more parts of oneself, and goes beyond what is already said and stated from the past, is crucial. The planet is worn out, unproductive, stagnant, and inactive when traditional, costume-like clothes are cloaked over human beings. They resemble the impoverishment of dull, negative states of mankind. Hopelessness and dullness occur when clothing is utilized to this degree.

Fashion as a language

The psychology of fashion is a part of making fashion healthy. There's an instinctual force of pattern in fashion that is psychological, and it leads to an evolved fashion language.

The intention and personal beliefs behind a person's way of dress is partly psychological. People are naturally drawn to fashion because it offers people a greater sense of vision.

Fashion isn't always taken seriously. As a form of communication, it's an underrated field of study. Yet fashion is a proven visual testament to the planet evolving. That alone makes it a noteworthy contribution. Fashion can be entertaining and light-hearted; however, it's narrow-minded to see fashion as an irrational, frivolous subject matter, for there is unquestionable depth to it.

Clothing is a daily symbol of life, and of the universe. Dressing is a sacred ritual like bathing, drinking, and eating. It is a sanctuary for the mind, body, and spirit. Wardrobes can actually provide more or equivalent healing effects than what other forms of therapy offer, when there is a recurring expansion of interconnection maintained through daily dressing.

We can look to clothing to better understand one another, to communicate with one another, because fashion is a language. Fashion exudes a force remedying a lack of understanding people and the world. No one is separate from fashion. Fashion is not separate from anything. Fashion is not an extension of nature, it is nature. Some of the more important aspects of life come into fruition when fashion communicates a reflection of existence.

There's a need to conceptualize fashion that is driven by psychological, physiological, and spiritual influences. For example, the concept of identifying and reflecting on our personal strengths and weaknesses in relation to our personal fashions intuitively harnesses a human/fashion connection. The simple act of dressing can help prompt triumphs over the endured trials of life.

Based on what is going on in a person's life internally, fashion disconnection can occur. A person doesn't always arrive at being comfortable in their own clothing or own skin. Clothing can become such a mirror of daily experiences that are not all comfortable. Having a connection between clothing and oneself eventually acts as a channel and an outlet. Clothing can then be a healing tool to decrease emotional suffering and physical pain. Fashion is a source of comfort and identity, consoling people when life situations and people cannot.

When personal style becomes negotiated, clothing becomes a mask, and this is not always an honest personal expression of self. The inner dialogue of a person's style can fluctuate between expressing false and true awareness. Clothing can be a false ideal when it doesn't reveal a person's true character or true spirit. Clothing can be a temporary escape rather than a mark of connection. This fashion escape may be needed at times, yet it can become a bit of a crutch.

Politics, media, and set, cultural standards put upon fashion can make one feel revulsion towards it. At certain points, fashion perceptions can lead a person to develop a distaste of others or of their own fashion. There can be a discouraging feeling when society, or oneself, uses fashion to fill voids and escape. This decreases the value of clothing.

It's good to have an undercurrent of rebellious inquisitiveness towards fashion, because this works to alter fashion views significantly. The fashion traps and guises, when observed, can prompt the revelations of fashion's deeper truths. These perceptive fashion observations are a search to find out that fashion has much more than it currently offers us. They opt to bring truths about in a person's wardrobe, conveying purposeful meaning and thoughtful inspiration.

The fashion archetype model: a modern fashion concept

True fashion archetypes versus false fashion stereotypes

Carl Jung, the Swiss psychiatrist, founded analytical psychology. He introduced the concept of "archetypes" as universal, archaic patterns of the collective unconscious. He theorized that humans represent one or several of the 12 major Jungian archetypes based on their psyche. Using the basis of Jung's archetype theory, I correlate specific fashion styles with the 12 archetype figures. I present this as the fashion archetype model, an evolved form of psychological, fashion communication. Transcending style through the psyche rooted in the Jungian archetypes presents a way of dress that accrues a deeper connection between people, society, and culture.

The fashion archetype model is psychologically driven. It is highly evolved on its course of connecting an individual's fashion identity to their psyche, for health. Rather than fashion perceived within the given stereotypes that numb the senses, the fashion archetype model bypasses and transcends stereotypical judgements found in fashion.

The fashion archetype model is made up of clothing styles that are in direct relation to the human psyche, making fashion a soulful endeavor when identified in this way. The 12 major archetype figures are: The Innocent, Sage, Explorer, Rebel, Magician, Hero, Lover, Jester, Everyman, Caregiver, Ruler, and Creator. All the above-mentioned archetype figures are honorable, representing the deeper aspects of the inner soul and spirit.

Carl Jung once said, "Thinking is difficult, that is why most people judge." This is the exact reason why we need the fashion archetype model, for a healthy psyche. Because we are automatically judging fashions when we stereotype them. Fashion stereotypes keep us from doing any further thinking about fashion, and keep us from its deeper purpose and meaning.

The major fashion stereotypes that create a minimal effect in the pursuit of fashion communication include: the jock, artist, punk, homeless, gangster, rock star, cowboy, yuppie, hippy, club-goer, *et cetera*. These labels can devalue our perception of style to a certain degree because stereotypes aren't being pursued perceptively and transcended in a mindful way. Fashion must go beyond the surface, and go beyond the meaning of fashion stereotypes.

The fashion archetype model ushers in a holistic approach of perceiving fashion, as it is more humane to perceive style archetypically than stereotypically. Perceiving style through the archetype model is much better for mental and emotional health. The fashion archetype model honors and respects a person's look without judgement, which is the opposite of how a fashion stereotype works, as they often create judgmental assumptions about a person.

The fashion archetype model is a remedy for the dated perception of viewing fashion as stereotypes that mask a person's true self. Plato links clothes with beauty, he said: "A beauty of fraudulent nature." That is to say, based on the clothes one wears, there is a distinct amount of masking, as well as a separation of the sense of self, creating judgement.

Archetype fashion is used as a force for the psyche to express itself. Labeling fashion with stereotypes is natural, but when fashion is not being interpreted in a mindful way, it disrupts the protective force field of the psyche and may cause a halt to the spiritual convictions of who a person is and is to become.

Fashion stereotype labeling makes fashion communication less advanced. They can hide people from revealing their true self, and they can make it hard for people to understand others. For example, if someone looks like a jock; when the word jock and the visual of what a jock looks like comes to mind, this stereotype label doesn't reveal the core of their psyche/identity.

Using the fashion archetype model, the jock stereotype is represented by the archetype figures: the leader, hero, adventurer, explorer, and the team player. These archetype figures symbolize humans as soulful, rather than if we were to simply label someone a stereotypical jock. Viewing a person as a jock often only measures the person's interest in sports, keeping fashion communication on the surface.

Clothing that resonates in ego form is stereotype fashion. Stereotype labels are biased, reflecting a limited mindset and an ego-based belief system. The opposite is the healthy, altruistic form of archetype fashion. We give power to ourselves and to those among us when we honor and respect fashion as archetype fashion. When a person has little to no ego, they are selfless and not in control, and a supernatural, divine force is.

A person's higher self is associated with practicing archetype fashion, versus the lower self that is stuck in a vicious cycle, practicing stereotype fashion. Practicing archetype fashion via the higher self attains a certain sense of recognizing one's own soul, and other people's soul through dress. When we stereotype fashion, it is depicted quickly without conscious thought. When people observe fashion and only see stereotypes, this is a generic way to identify fashion. It does not get at the root of who a person truly is or how authentic a person can be identified as.

Stereotypes create false awareness because it is a lack of viewing dress as a tool for nurturing the innermost self. The psyche is gently treated when perceiving fashion through the fashion archetypes. It fosters confidence, positivity, and self-assurance, adding a sense of worth and esteem effectively.

Archetype fashion does not control like stereotype fashion does. It cultivates the need to feel and express the inner psyche. Labeling a person as a stereotype based on their style disrupts evolved thinking. Archetype fashion leads to a deeper connection to life and humanity. To see a person's spirit and soul through fashion, and/or looking past the clothed body, is better. Clothing needs to serve the purpose of understanding humans in a meaningful way.

Archetype fashion leads to positive reinforcements of a

person's worth, it supports personal development, and honors a person's soul path. It's about an appreciation of clothing, and valuing one's respective traits, actions, behavior, and mindset behind their personal style.

The negative aspects of fashion stereotypes

When dress is viewed and observed through the modern Jungian archetypes, there's less interest in labeling fashion stereotypically. Stereotyping fashion produces false awareness, as society is programmed to typically view stereotypes in a compartmentalized, egotistical way. They can breed an on-the-surface, shallow mentality and narrow thinking. People can feel pressured and pigeonholed within the practice of generically stereotyping fashion. It negligently limits perspective, and diminishes the profound importance of fashion psychology and fashion's mode of communication. A stereotyped label increases the chances that a person will judge others, disapprove of them, and segregate from them.

Throughout the generations there's been an aggressive demonstration of importance to stereotype a person based on their style. Just look to the Victorian age when purple-colored fabrics were only worn by the wealthy. The purple color was used for power and control. Purple was used as a status symbol that prided itself in egotism. Clothing designed to specifically cater to low, middle, and upper classes can be considered as stereotyping fashion.

The agenda of stereotyping fashion instills false values of a false fashion system, and it has overruled the healthy, authentic, fashion archetype model. It has blocked the mind-expansive archetypes of a person's style, stunting the growth of perceiving style in an evolutionary way. Stereotypes distract people from the truth, narrowing a person's perceptions to the degree that when associating with fashion, it can become a burden.

Stereotypes can lead to false connotations of style. Style

becomes desensitized when dress is minimized to false fashion stereotypes. Stereotyping fashion can be a bit of a mockery against fashion with the potential to breed ignorance overall, creating a lack of inner soul reflection.

In order to transform stereotype labeling and create positive interpretations of dress, we must actualize a higher power to intervene and to move us towards the authentic fashion archetype model.

In order to bypass fashion stereotypes, we need to use the fashion archetype model

Listed below are the 12 Jungian archetypes that represent and depict the larger picture of style perception. There are several fashion stereotypes and styles by genre listed with each archetype. This is in order to detect and transcend limited fashion perceptions. It is for the higher purpose of identifying fashion with the psyche, and transcending the fashion stereotypes that have limited, psychological value.

Apart from the fashion archetypes, using the term "style genres" or "fashion styles" to replace "fashion stereotypes" is a preferred way of labeling fashions. Yet style genres are most usually framed as stereotypes, and they still describe fashion in a less perceptive way. Style genres can be transcended further and be associated with a deeper meaning through the fashion archetypes. Fashion archetypes of clothing speak a broader and deeper form of fashion communication.

There are numerous ways to learn about how specified style genres can be transcended into the archetype figures. Because the archetype model is flexible, it gives an individual the opportunity to identify with archetype fashion and stereotype fashion in their own way, through their own perceptions and experiences.

Listed below are the dominating traits of each Jungian archetype. This is to prepare and root the fashion archetypes for further revelations via personal reflection, and deepening fashion identification on the soul/psyche level. This is for the cause of opening new fashion perspectives of fashion psychology. We all have every archetype within; it is a matter of connecting with all of them, and some more strongly than others in different moments in time, and using them as a form of fashion communication and self-expression in a healthy, positive way.

The 12 archetypes; their traits and the style genres associated with them:

The spiritual person

Innocent: (safety) The Innocent is optimistic, and tends to believe things should naturally go well in life. They enjoy dreaming. They seem drawn to the good in people. They enjoy keeping faith. *Style genre*: Hippy, Youthful, Earthy, Artsy, Whimsical, Folkloric

Sage: (knowledge) The Sage is one who is of wisdom, knowledge, and power. The Sage is reckoned to be a part of the spiritual side of one's personality via the unconscious. *Style genre*: Mystical, Bohemian, Exotic, Avant-garde, Baroque, Tribal

Explorer: (freedom) The Explorer is an adventurer and one who wants to discover the world. They are courageous, independent, and inspired. *Style genre*: The Outdoorsman, Hiker, Tomboy, Skater, Surfer, Indie, Rustic

The person who leaves a mark

Rebel: (liberation) The Rebel is one who speaks out against discrimination and injustice, and doesn't conform to trends. The Rebel likes to take the road less traveled. *Style genre*: Punk, Rocker, Cowgirl/Cowboy, Grunge, Heavy-Metal

Magician: (power) The Magician is associated with power, alchemy, and transformation. The magician is a free-thinker and a visionary. *Style genre*: Fairy/Wizard, Mythological, Futuristic, Space Age, Sci-Fi

Hero: (mastery) The Hero is one who has overcome obstacles and possesses the interest and ability to achieve ambitious goals. They are associated with attaining the elixir of life. *Style genre*: Athletic, Sporty, Military, Supernatural

The person who connects with others

Lover: (intimacy) The Lover is passionate and wants close relationships, and to achieve intimacy. The Lover enjoys making people feel special. *Style genre*: Romantic, Retro, Vintage, Clubber, Dapper, Elegant, Formal

Jester: (pleasure) Also known as a trickster or comedian. The Jester likes to entertain and appreciate the happiness in life. The Jester enjoys being playful and light-hearted, and is not afraid to go against the rules. *Style genre*: Gangster, Hip-Hop, Flamboyant, Steampunk, Vibrant, Eclectic

Everyman: (belonging) The Everyman enjoys being a part of a group or activity. They value other people. Part of their purpose is to be accepted by others and to belong. They are friendly and want to do good in the world and to be a part of something. *Style genre*: Preppy, Chic, Classic, Professional, Modest, Androgyny, Conventional Fads, Traditional

The person who provides structure

Caregiver: (service) Caregivers have a sense of selflessness. They enjoy helping others. They are generous, compassionate, and eager to provide as it becomes a reward for themselves. *Style genre*: Maternal/Paternal, Maternity, Girl Next Door/Guy Next Door

Ruler: (control) The Ruler likes to be the leader and in control. They are interested in safety and security. They are role models that enjoy being in power. *Style genre*:

Ceremonial, New Age, Formal, Sophisticated, Aristocrat, High Priest/Priestess

Creator: (innovation) The Creator is a non-conformist, visionary, and genuine. They enjoy being intuitively creative, and they like to make things happen. They like to foster new ideas and are enlightened. *Style genre*: Trend-Driven, Casual, Minimalist, Non-Traditional, Edgy, Athleisure

The evolution of fashion archetypes

To fully actualize the fashion archetype model's potential, multiple archetypes need to be expressed and made visible within a look. A person has multiple archetype figures that represent him or her. No one is limited to expressing one dominant trait. It is healthy to wear multiple fashion archetype styles and even merge multiple archetype styles together. However, there can also be an exploitation of power, if a person is wearing all different types of fashion styles to claim ownership over these styles. This can become a form of control and mask who a person truly is when we aim to own fashion. It's also a form of fashion theft. There is a fine line. Furthermore, we don't really want to mask ourselves with fashion genres, we want to embrace and express ourselves through them.

Multiple fashion archetype styles need to merge and blend within a look. If a style is overtly dominant to one specific archetype, additional design elements of a fashion design can be added to balance out over-dominating behaviors of a style, whether it be through yin/yang balance, four element fashion, or other means. Also, styles that correlate with the fashion archetype figures are much broader than fixed stereotype styles.

Perceiving fashion by stereotype provides a lack of grounding. Personality traits become obscured and muddled.

Stereotyping fashion can limit a person's story, expression, and livelihood. It pushes people towards the ego model of ownership and control in fashion. It doesn't allow the surrendering of oneself in the way that fashion archetype dress does. The perplexing fashion misperceptions caused by stereotyping fashion will phase out as fashion evolves.

Wearing specific types of dress may create segregation between different people's wardrobes and lifestyles to a certain degree. This cannot always be changed as there are prominent archetype styles involved in a person's individual wardrobe that need to be expressed, as people do have dominant archetype figures in their psyche displayed through their wardrobe. The dominant traits of a specified archetype are naturally expressed through personal style. A person's dominant archetypes do change and fluctuate throughout a person's life and in the moment, however.

The Innocent fashion archetype versus the hippy stereotype in fashion

Included here is an extensive breakdown and an example of the Innocent fashion archetype, typically viewed as the hippy fashion stereotype. The fashion archetype that counteracts the "hippy" fashion stereotype is the Innocent archetype. The hippy stereotype works as a controlled fashion mechanism. Observing a person's fashion, and associating them with the Innocent fashion archetype rather than the hippy stereotype is a positive reinforcement. We are naturally going to immediately view a person's style stereotypically, as it has been ingrained in us to do so, but the conscious approach is to go beyond fashion stereotypes.

Recognizing the Innocent archetype in a style rather than the hippy stereotype leads to further thinking and personal empowerment for both the wearer and viewer. It provides intrigue and insightfulness. The Innocent archetype figure is a free spirit, full of faith, optimistic. Traits of the Innocent archetype figure are that they feel a sense of wonderment, and they are a dreamer. The Innocent archetype expresses happiness, youthfulness, a sense of feeling alive. All of these qualities are sacred.

Perceiving a person's style and personality as an expression of the Innocent archetype is much more humane than denoting a person as a hippy. Thinking they are a hippy could create all kinds of negative incentives of fashion that mislead the soul-character of a person. It makes no difference if we see a person's style and think "hippy," it's the act of consciously looking past the stereotypical label in order to perceive the soul identity of a person through fashion.

The term "hippy" can be manipulatively and derogatively used. In any case, the term "bohemian" is a healthier term to use for representing hippy style, and bohemian style can be looked at as more of a style genre than a stereotype. The term "hippy" can be negatively associated with labels such as a crazy artist, druggy, or an unkempt lethargic person. This explains the degrees of aggression towards fashion stereotype labels which are not typically discussed. They need to be addressed to provide resolution and a psychological transition to healthier ways of perceiving humans and their fashions. This is out of respect and honor of a person's soul.

Viewing hippy style as Innocent style makes the observer have a better reflection and understanding as to why this style exists. Archetype fashion creates useful boundaries as well, because there can be an issue with styles becoming a controlling, power-trip endeavor.

Any stereotype can potentially form a power play, because a person dressed in a certain stereotype can be seen as being above others, or above other stereotypes, even if the wearer doesn't realize that is happening. The hippy style can be associated with a class that is liberal, far-out, and otherworldly in terms of beliefs and behaviors. They march to the beat of their own drum and can be associated with the pursuit of a higher calling. It's a privilege to be all these things, but not in the context of the belief that they feel superior.

Due to style stereotypes being a form of segregation, in some cases, if a person sees qualities of the hippy stereotype in another person's outfit, the observer may unconsciously feel rejection and revolt against these same qualities within themselves if they don't wear that particular hippy style. Psychologically, if the observer sees the hippy style but does not dress like a hippy themselves, the hippy style can potentially push away the viewer's personal access to the traits of the universal Innocent archetype. It can lead to a feeling of emptiness. It can also create ideas that the traits of specific styles are exclusive to certain people.

Unconsciously a wearer may embrace ownership of particular dominant traits in a given style, but they wish they could wear those styles others do. For example, a person may have an unconscious or conscious belief, thinking that: "I am not a hippy because I don't wear hippy fashions, and therefore I don't have that 'hippy' personality, they do." They may also think: "I do not dress like a hippy. Therefore, the hippy has something I don't."

It is as if parts of the self, parts of the soul and spirit, are not being clearly expressed within one's personal style and are being primarily admired through another person's style. This may cause a person to feel unwanted emotions. This can fuel envy and create a feeling of lack in the viewer. It's a power-interested game and an unconscious mode of operation built from an ego-based system of fashion.

Viewing and observing the Innocent archetype style as the hippy style stereotype, it can demonstrate unwanted control and power negligently over these traits. Stereotype labels can also become a power trip. They can become used as a manipulation tactic. When a feeling of ownership is present over a stereotype it can make others feel they are not of those qualities if they don't dress that way. Fashion should be an open invitation, not an invitation-only. Fashion should reflect a resemblance of equality, naturally gravitating towards balance through the fashion archetypes.

By choosing not to dress in the hippy style, it doesn't mean people are separate from those common qualities or traits associated with it. These traits and qualities of the Innocent archetype are channeled through other styles and other archetypes effectively. Additionally, choosing to wear another style doesn't limit the variation of fashion archetype qualities that specific style represents. Archetype traits are expressed among a range of styles on a broad scale.

Generally speaking, stereotyping fashion can become a sport and a game of human competition. Embracing one's own and others' archetype figures provides an opportunity to develop core strengths that support the psyche, not deflect it. Archetype fashion is a solution, giving us more opportunity to relate to these very qualities within ourselves, as much as valuing these qualities in another person.

Psychologically and energetically, fashion and style are stemmed from the traits of the psyche, and they can be intentionally or unintentionally stolen from other people through style. Also, styles conflicting with others' styles can become an ego transmission, and can disrespect other people's individual expression indirectly.

It is easy to judge and make assumptions about a person by the way they dress. If a person doesn't dress in a hippy style they would naturally not be labeled as a hippy. This is how powerful and communicative fashion can be. Yet our approach to fashion needs to become an introspective process. Fashion needs to be further examined for the health of the psyche. Fashion showcases communicatively, but because of what the programmed society says, fashion can also divert people from the truth. Archetype fashion is a demonstration of the truth of who a person is.

Fashion in performance art

Fashion is a form of communication and a language of its own in theater, film, and the ballet. Clothing used in the performing arts conjures symbolism, poetic expression, and abstract thinking. Clothing in theater is fashion performing. "Fashion performing" is used to convey words and emotions that cannot necessarily be literally spoken about, but are seen and felt, provoking thought. It gives us an opportunity to view fashion in a new light.

The concept of clothing as its own entity can produce a method of relating to fashion in a deeper way. Fashion performing is clothing that becomes a piece of action, not only a piece of material. It is used as an artistic vehicle, and a moving channel similar to any other form of art medium. A garment that emphasizes a mood, a role, a reaction, and a mental idea initiates a feeling and a story of its own. Fashion used as a prop can certainly turn itself into words, symbols, poetry, and can offer ideas and inspiration.

Fabrics and costumes that perform with and through the performer reveal that the relationship we have with clothing can become a symbolic extension of who a person is and it can showcase their story, rather than it be just a piece of material covering the body. A performer's costume represents an eternal pattern of the performance. The connection is deep due to the fact that apparel is placed directly over the skin's surface, so it belongs to us.

Costume directly participates actively in a performance, and initiates a performance, as well. This can be found in the way the fabrics and designs of costumes are deliberately or unconsciously expressed. For example, a costume can be worn effectively to convey a message as it moves or interacts with the body in order to communicate to the wearer and viewer. The fashion/body connection of costume creates a symphony, an orchestra, and reveals a fulfilling union between self and clothing.

Fashion performing may appear as an abstract concept, but it is part of an effort to make people become aware of the multiple fashion perspectives, and reveal the purpose behind fashion that therapeutically treats the body. When clothing is performing, it symbolically reveals the soul and our connection with the expansiveness of the universe.

Sometimes there's a struggle when a garment doesn't feel perfect on. Yet one is constantly striving for the feeling of solution through fashion. Through fashion exploration, we perceive fashion as not only material but as a part of faith, like a heart worn on the sleeve, and as a story that can open up new opportunities that make fashion sacred.

When the body is naked, something is missing and it's not just the cloth. Fashion is our protection, and dressing is a divine activity that keeps one in tune with the reason why we are here on planet Earth. When we use fashion as a way to break any barriers we have with the concept of dress and of life, it forms a reason to reconcile with fashion.

Effects of costume and its form of communication

Ballet costume has the ability to tell a story. The modern costume designs presented in the Triadic Ballet by Oscar Schlemmer, from 1922, completely defy common dance costume. Schlemmer was a painter, designer, sculptor, and choreographer.

The costumes of the Triadic Ballet extend themselves to philosophical thinking. Schlemmer's work was meant to be perceived as philosophical. His costume designs were a moving portrayal that declared philosophical statements about human existence.

The costumes designed by Schlemmer himself are incredibly signature and defy nature. The cylinder, sphere, cone, spiral, and other geometric shapes were used to bring Schlemmer's brilliant designs to life. They are bizarre, to the point where they redefined what costume is. They are a verbal, visual, stylish poetry.

When fashion performs, language barriers cease to exist. The costumes themselves can create a heightened state of awareness that even proceeds to answer existential questions like: "What is life?" In the grand scheme of things, costume designs can communicate theoretical fashion information to the viewer. Fashion becomes a force, and a value that does not define life, but honestly questions its mystery and proceeds to answer it.

Chapter 3

Healthy Fashion for the Emotional and Energetic Body

Healthy fashion supports the emotional body

Fashion plays an important role for the emotional body on a physiological and metaphysical level. Fashion is in support of the energy body, which affects the emotional body, because emotions are made up of energy. Fashion can be used as a tool to integrate human emotions within the mental, physical, spiritual, and energetic bodies.

There's an art and science to working with one's emotions through the wardrobe. There is a symbiotic effect happening between the clothing a person wears and the body's natural activity of purging and releasing emotions and toxic energies. Clothing naturally absorbs a person's emotions and toxic energy throughout the day. It can establish more balanced moods and dissolve toxic emotions as they arise. This occurs naturally.

Emotions play a large role in life. Emotions are made up of energy. *Emotere*, a Latin root of the word "emotion," means energy in motion. Rather than emotions being circulated and stuck within the body, clothing naturally acts as a tool, filtering and neutralizing emotions. Fabric can then hold onto these emotions, especially in the first and second layers of an outfit.

Dirty garments don't need to have an odor or stain to demonstrate their need of being laundered. Clothing can feel and be energetically mucky after wear, and this is caused by the accumulating energies and emotions that are released into them throughout the day. Laundering and other methods like refolding, steaming, and pressing a garment remove and lift the unwanted energy of residual emotions that naturally accumulate in fabric. Also, burning sage, cedarwood, and sweetgrass, or spraying water mixed with essential oils directly onto the garments can release the stuck-on energy.

Fabrics are like crystals, acting as an antenna of energy. Like crystals, they are constantly absorbing, transmuting, and neutralizing negative energy. They collect and clear out negative energies. Synthetic fabrics typically do not have energy transfer capabilities like plant-based fabrics do.

Plant-based fabrics are pliable and have vitality; synthetic fabrics are static and remote. Synthetic materials are not structurally built like the crystalline structure of plant-based fabrics. Crystals contain a crystal lattice which is also found in plant-based fibers. In quantum physics, crystals are treated as piezoelectric, they generate an electric charge. It's the electric polarization that produces a healing response.

Over time, a human's energy output creates wear on clothing. Humans give off an energy, mostly an electromagnetic radiation. A resting human gives off about 100–125 watts of energy. Clothing has its own energy cycle. There's a point in time when a garment needs to be taken to a thrift store or thrown out based on a person's energy output on the material. It's not only the holes, tattered parts of clothing, rips, and tears that make a piece of clothing ready to be thrown away or given up. The daily, emotional release of human energy production puts wear on clothing, as well. It is not always visible to the eye, but it is felt.

A garment may no longer resonate with the wearer's energy after a person has put a lot of use into the garment. However, based on the technical design of fabric, and the garment's design, it can have life left for another person to wear it. A garment can be regenerated for someone else. Some pieces need to be passed over, while other garments still have energetic value to another wearer down the road.

How is this so? The reason for this is that clothing can become renewed, refreshed, and made new by another person's energetic composition. This is based on the individual's energy body and its likeness and attraction to the used garment's fabric and design. Additionally, if the garment is recycled and made into a new, regenerated fabric, this revamps the fabric for more, continued use, displaying the same energetic properties as it did when the fabric was new.

Clothing can be used predominantly as an emotional outlet, and to safely release emotions. Fashion can grant us spiritual and emotional resolution from senseless conflict with oneself and others because daily attire initiates and produces a physical, mental, emotional, and energetic release. Furthermore, it can also protect us from unwanted emotions. Certain outfits act as a protective layer which can then offer more balanced moods, as they ward off internal and external, negative emotions and/ or stimuli. This form of protective barrier is a fashion healing modality.

Negative energies are attracted to stained, torn, holed, ripped clothing, and they tend to cling to them. There are exceptions, like if they are designed that way, and are supposed to appear as an artistic design element, or if a garment is simply loved, there is a difference. The attachment of loving a garment is healthy because the soul and spirit desires it. But there's a letting-go point. It's a freeing feeling to throw away clothing, and doing this can energetically cut ties to emotions and memories that no longer need to be held on to.

Negative energy and evil-like influences in clothing that affect the emotional body

Styles can be negative in disguise. It could be a basic white tee shirt or a mock, blood-stained ritual shirt, its negative vibration is not always noticeable, yet it can be felt. It gets down to the frequency of the fabric, as some hold a negative vibration. Also, a person's own energy body can negatively affect the garment.

Possessed fashion can really disturb the emotional body. An obvious example is a piece of clothing with a satanic symbol on it. This symbol is not just a "symbol," it can be used to perform satanic activity. Possessed fashion can look haunting and fear-driven. This can even create negative feelings and negative emotions.

Take a voodoo doll as an example. Voodoo dolls are made up of materials, but there's so much more to it than a doll made of fabrics, trims, and stuffing material. The design of the doll can also contribute to it being evil. When the doll becomes possessed with evil from the spells and curses being attached to it, this is where the materials and objects are affected. The objects and materials can hold a negative vibration or "curse."

Some of the traits and symptoms of possessed clothing include these: It may be uncomfortable to wear. It can also unconsciously be bothersome. If it just feels off, like something is wrong with the fabric or design, that is also an immediate indicator. With possessed clothing, there could be a negative symbol or a very heavy, negative energetic feeling of the fabric and design in its appearance.

Whether a garment is soiled with permanent stains, or a garment has frayed pant hems that drag in the dirt, the energy will be off. Attracting negative vibrations can be caused if a person has an imbalanced electromagnetic body. Being aware of the electromagnetic systems can help one find out if a garment or their body is electromagnetically balanced or not.

Evil-based clothing harbors stuck energy because the mechanics of a fabric can be portal-like. So, a garment can then become either a portal for sluggish, distorted, bad energy or a portal for healthy, positive energy. When evil or negative energy is transferred through clothing it can hold a person in a state of ill-effects.

People who are drawn to low-vibration clothing are not always in complete recognition that they are attracting a low-vibration garment, or that they can attract or repel negativity via apparel. Some people, however, embrace evil-like clothing as a symbol of their interests, because it's their intention to possess an evil-influenced identity. However, clothing is a means of soul reflection but not always an accurate portrayal of it. Styles can be a fleeting phase, not always a complete soul-expression.

Some people dress for self-punishment. This is a form of an attack on oneself. Self-punishment through fashion is partially associated with past traumas. Whatever abusive, traumatic situation a person has been in, clothing can be used as a negative tool to express negative behaviors and actions towards oneself that were created by past traumas.

People can suffer in a negative life-cycle which can be expressed through their fashion. For example, it's sometimes tempting to wear clothes that look good yet feel very uncomfortable. This is a sacrifice, however. Psychologically, people are able to become numb to the feeling of pain. A person then becomes immune to negative clothing. Sacrificing ourselves in the name of fashion is not as innocent as it sounds.

Outfits have the ability to control or liberate us. Oftentimes fashion doesn't agree with us. A bad outfit can endorse a bad day, debilitating it to some degree. Sometimes, no matter what is worn, we may not feel good in it, and this might simply happen, because we may occasionally need bad-tasting fashion, just as there is a need for the occasional bad mood. Sometimes it can be easier to blend in, and wear clothes that appease social regimes that have been placed on society. Everyone wants to feel accepted.

The root of various ailments can be eased by fashion design and personal style. From physical injury to emotional suffering, people naturally gravitate to fashion that soothes and protects.

Some outfits can cause disruption and problems, while other outfits can make a person feel content and satisfied. Fashion, essentially, can alleviate a negative condition.

Choosing positive clothing is an opportunity, an invitation to have high spirits. When we seek out the wisdom of fashion more and more, in a deeper way, there's a series of mental and emotional forces that divinely intervene, and help narrate our choices of fashion. This is a form of spiritual intervention.

Fashion and textiles as visual art

Aesthetically pleasing, visually artistic fashion is a window to the world of wellness and healing. There's an initiation that comes about when fashion and art are combined. Together, they work as a therapeutic, healing component for mental and emotional wellbeing.

Art is an innovative invention of creativity expressed. It uses the human imagination and life-force. It's a superior form of intelligence that holds power. Clothing infused with artistic creativity can speak very powerfully. When more energy and concentration is behind artistic fashion, it substantially produces more creative power.

Fashion designs made to look like visual art are creative channels, offering sustenance to a person's soul. Artistic fashion is like a prescription, enabling society to leap out of the crux of pain. Pain can age people. Art is definitely an important part of fashion, and helps people stay youthful. To become or stay youthful, constant newness in fashion and art is necessary.

The arts and healthcare industries use visual art to heal and psychologically support one's mental health. Visual art expressed in fashion design eases anxiety, emotional suffering, and depression. It can have a stimulating, soothing, inspiring effect, supporting people's everyday existence.

Fashion and art combined bring our emotional intelligence

to the forefront. Art is proven to evoke emotion and feelings. It stimulates and revitalizes the mind by provoking thought. Part of art's primary mode of operation is to activate the left and right parts of the brain.

Visual imagery as an unlimited healing and therapeutic opportunity is vast. It can be from a fabric's color, pattern, or texture. As an example, nature-inspired visual design is healing, because the body's biological rhythm is quite similar to the rhythms found in nature. So, visual designs imitating nature are therapeutic.

Art reduces cortisol, the stress-hormone. Being creative and wearing artistic fashion that expresses creativity releases endorphins that will help reduce pain. Additionally, fashion can be used as a form of meditation. That is partly what fashion is for, to bring a form of awareness to focus. One is constantly surrounded by images, moving a person into negative or positive states of mind. While there may be stress throughout the day, positive, artistic, visual imagery in fashion can enhance and even make a person's day more therapeutically meditative.

Wearing visual art can be a form of inspiration, similar to the feelings and inspiration that come about when viewing art at a museum or art gallery. Art museums attract millions of visitors per year. People are moved emotionally and are intellectually inspired from their own personal impressions when observing and interacting with visual art.

Fashion on the street is a form of visual art. Street fashion is meaningful on an emotional, mental, and spiritual level. Bill Cunningham was a famous fashion photographer and hat designer from NYC. He celebrated street fashion. His fashion photography reveals the special, creative aspects of fashion, and he revealed synchronistic patterns found in fashion. These synchronistic patterns were trends he would find on the streets.

Street fashion communicates both artistically and multidimensionally. Street fashion is a true inspiration. Fashion is not only a product for function and beautification; it's also a gift that is shared and given from people walking by on the street. It's a lift for people.

Fashion therapy is a healing tool similar to art therapy. Fashion therapy is not just shopping therapy; however, shopping and selecting garments is a major factor conducive to the healing process. Fashion as visual art is a healing therapy, a tool to connect with the intrinsic self. It is part of fashion as a language, and it is revealed to those using fashion as a visual aid. People who have their own artistic expression, and understand the importance of their individual, evolutionary fashion process, they know the value of human growth and personal power through the creative use of their fashion and way of dress.

Dressing is a creative activity

Personal style is a statement of creative freedom. It can reveal the power of a person. The spiritual, creative power in fashion, and the art of dressing is partly made up of the beauty and emotion that is found in art. Fashion as art is appreciated for its beauty and emotional power. Beauty and emotion combined can become an "Aha!" moment. A fashion look can become a part of one's being, creating an opportunity to reflect and recognize that we are all a part of something bigger than ourselves.

Creativity and artistic pursuits naturally influence a way a person dresses, too, as fashion can also be viewed as a form of creating art. Dressing is an art. It's a creative process marked by story and theme that fuels a person's style. Artistic fashion transforms an ever-changing wardrobe through symbolism, poeticism, and the therapeutic elements of fashion design. Like the words and thoughts translated through poetry, these same words and thoughts can be represented symbolically in fashion.

Poetic fashion is definitely a fashion therapy technique. Creating and finding this poetic connection in fashion design and style can be created and found through symbolism in dress, by its color, shape, texture, silhouette, pattern, and line. All these design elements can create a patterned sequence, which are often found and expressed in poems, or in a musical composition.

Another way to establish a deeper connection with fashion is to use it as an introspective journaling activity. Over time, this intention of documenting looks daily or weekly supports a more balanced mood, and works to spark creativity. Daily outfits don't have to be documented in a fashion journal for it to work therapeutically. It still works if the looks aren't actually documented either through photos or written down. It can be an unplanned, improvisational, undocumented fashion journal experience. Reviewing and reflecting on our own daily looks is a health benefit. It's a personal testament of life's existence.

Fashion is storytelling. People go through many style phases, and they all showcase many different attitudes, behaviors, stories, and soul growth. Style evolution persists to help people figure out their own identity and who they are on deeper levels. Everyone conquers time cycles of trends, and captures fashion milestones through their ever-changing wardrobes. The soul, as it goes through the fashion cycles, this creates a soul's evolutionary growth. This can be looked at as a form of achievement.

Fashion memories, reflecting on them, can be a fashion therapy. For instance, reflecting on a fashion memory of a specific look, like if a person predominantly wears a grey sweater and skinny jeans for a whole season. Reflecting on this, this outfit may be creating stagnancy. However, through analyzing the look, it's noticeable this look is not always a static expression but a canvas of opportunity.

This grey sweater and skinny jean look, when worn rather religiously, is a reflection of an incubatory phase in life. Also, at the same time, the look moves like all changing styles do. It can give a sense of security and stability, becoming a grounding embodiment, not a short-term fashion trend pursuit. Between a museum or an art gallery, the outfit is portrayed as the museum with its longer "style" life cycle.

Each day, this persistent, daily look can give a person a renewed feeling. It can tell a new story every day, yet also give a feeling of nostalgia that proves to be comforting. Dress is a daily invitation to feel remarkably connected to our personal growth and wellbeing.

High fashion as an art

Societies of all classes can respect and admire the devotional use of fashion identified as an art. It is evident that there are revelations of fashion being used as a source of power. Fashion is also a source to feel protected. You will find that styles and fashions may be random, yet there's a deep connection between humans, and fashion as an art. It's also visibly marked on the behaviors and attitudes which people have with their clothes. Naturally improvising with fashion looks exerts a kind of creative power behind fashion, and makes fashion an art.

Looking closely, people are some of the most fashionable when they're not only driven by necessity between clothing and self, they also have a real need and respect between themselves and their clothing used as a creative expression. It doesn't matter what it looks like; it's about the feeling and representation of a person's style. However temporary or long-term an outfit may be, fashion as an art is soulful fashion embraced.

Most people are genuinely highly creative. They utilize clothes as a creative channel. This creativity stems from improvisational skills partly based on using fashion as a significant form of communication. Depending on a person's need of survival and their practical use of fashion, some people may feel they look unstylish, yet it is still an art form, and others feel drawn to their clothes as a form of real, high style.

Some people have a profound way of utilizing fashion for purpose. There's a finite, artistic force and a divinely timed synchronistic exactness to style and dress. Clothing is typically a possession they own, becoming a prized resource for their soul and general wellbeing. Garments are divinely chosen and sometimes out of their complete control. An artistic wardrobe can be looked at as a form of surrender when divine consciousness intervenes.

By grace, people find their clothing via divine timing. The connection between clothing and the human being becomes strong. Without a doubt, everyone can be inspired by fashion, because there's a specific source of creativity that is expressed through the wardrobe, and, in a sense, a person can reveal fashion's holiness.

Color therapy in fashion

Color therapy, also known as chromotherapy, is the science of using colors and their frequencies to adjust body vibrations for health. It is a therapeutic science used for thousands of years, originating in Egypt, India, Native America, and Tibet. There's a constant interaction between humans and colors. We just have to look around us to see hundreds of different colors working to support us. The colors all around us provide an energy transaction that works to treat the body, mind, and spirit.

An example of using color to treat the body: Egyptians built solarium rooms. They are light-filled rooms of a specific tinted, colored light for curing disease and healing injury. They used a variety of colors to perform healing based on particular ailments. Color light therapy is not the only way to receive healing from color. The dye colors in fabric do the same thing. Fabrics act as the carrier of a color's vibration.

Color is vibrating light. Doctors use phototherapy (light therapy), a blue light as a treatment for hyperbilirubinemia and jaundice. Yellow color can lift depression. Blue color has been found to cure anxiety. Color can support the physical body, elevate mood, and can also increase energy.

Hanna Kroeger, the master herbalist and renowned healer, told her patients to lie in bed and sleep with a red and green towel placed above and/or below them. The colors' frequency would then heal the body overnight. This can be achieved also during the daytime through our daily attire.

Colors are attuned to specific frequencies. Color variation is needed because of the differing wavelengths of each color. The colors' differing wavelengths respond to the organs, glands, the human energy field, as well as human's mental and emotional states. Each color has unique therapeutic value to support the variation of ailments a person may have. Scientists say the body needs light as it is a nutrient for health. Color is nutrition for the human energy field. Use of color variation is likened to the way we need several different nutrients, vitamins, and minerals.

The body is organic living matter made up of 100 trillion cells energetically vibrating. Color is light moving, and is absorbed directly into body cells. The mitochondria and DNA of the human body needs specific color wavelengths of light. Light transmitted into body cells opens up new channels of healing for the body.

Wearing color can support the body's chakras and unblock stagnant energy. Colors can create grounding and spiritually light, lifted emotions for a person by its characteristics. Color is associated with spiritual consciousness. If it was brought to the attention of the public more, that the color of fabrics has a medicinal effect, this world would be less sick.

Healthy fashion for the energy body: the frequency and vibration of fabrics and textile dyes

We appear as dense physical beings, yet the body is merely energy materialized. The frequencies of a human's physical body and energy body need to collaborate and coexist with the frequencies of clothing. Fabrics are made of energy matter. The atomic particles of plant-based fibers are constantly moving and altering as time goes on. A fabric's frequency is never static. Based on varying factors, a fabric's frequency can be naturally altered or unnaturally manipulated.

The renowned engineer and scientist, Nikola Tesla, once said, "If you want to find the secrets of the universe, think in terms of energy, frequency, and vibration." It is natural for the mind and body to become in tune with the energetic forces of the universe. Frequency can be noticed and felt perceptually. There is a spiritual essence in frequency. A fabric's electrical, energetic, magnetic component is spiritual; it is not just scientific.

The color, design, and frequency of attire create something that's similar to a musical composition. There are varying types of frequency, tones, and notes within a piece of classical music just like there are varying types of frequency, tones and notes in a fashion design. Clothing constantly vibrates, resulting in a musical synthesis of vibrational frequency.

Fashion designs, fabrics, and dyes of the highest vibrational frequency are the healthiest. There are different ways of measuring frequency for its value, and many of these methods we have yet to discover and develop. Some frequencies are toxic, negative, unbalanced, with a low vibration.

Electromagnetic frequencies (EMFs), radio waves, cellphone towers, nuclear power plants, and electrical power plants are examples of unbalanced, negative "low" frequency. Calling their frequencies "low" does not describe the "speed" of their frequencies. Low is linked to its toxicity and negativity.

Most synthetic fabrics do not have a "high" or "healthy" vibration because of the type of ingredients and chemicals used to make them. Because many of these chemicals are toxic, the chemical composition of synthetic fabrics, its vibration and frequency is most likely disturbed. A vibration cannot be pure or considered "high" if the chemicals used are toxic or carcinogenic, especially if they are combined with other harsh chemicals found in fabrics and fabric dyes. The frequency of many synthetic fabrics, more and more, will go against the grain of a body's natural frequency.

However, the body is able to transmute negative frequencies of synthetic fabrics, it has a natural ability to do so. For example, if synthetic fabrics and synthetic dyes have ergonomic properties, such as the fabrics' dye colors that give healing effects, or if they are incredibly soft and comfortable fabrics, some of their "low vibration" and negative qualities can become transmuted and they will be therapeutic, and not have such an extreme, negative effect on a person.

In order to make a discernment about whether a garment or fabric is negative, take a polluted swamp and its disrupted, disturbed frequency versus an invigorating, unpolluted ocean. The frequency of the low-vibrating, polluted swamp becomes a death portal with no high-energetic frequency. Energy blocks and negative frequency as well as neutralization of the body's energetic channels can occur. By contrast, the ocean with its salty water is buzzing, the waves are swirling, its currents create vital energy and it is a portal of positivity.

A way to find out whether a fabric is healthy or unhealthy is by the use of the pendulum. The Native American Indians would find their plant medicine with a sacred stick, or pendulum. A pendulum is a supernatural tool, but it is also scientific. "The rod, the reed, and the staff," also named the "divining rod," is mentioned in the Bible, so the pendulum is not evil. It is the way it could be used that would make it harmful, because it is not supposed to be used to predict things, it is supposed to be used to find out whether something is healthy or unhealthy for someone.

Typically, when the pendulum is placed over the fabric, if the pendulum swings right, or clockwise, that means "yes," or "positive." If it swings left, or counterclockwise, it means "no," or "unhealthy." The master herbalist and healer Reverend Hanna Kroeger wrote "The Pendulum Book." It explains how the pendulum works, and how to use the pendulum.

Fashion and the frequency of the heart

Wearing fashion in correlation with the heart promotes health. Clothing must resonate with the heart, as the body and mind revolves around it. Everything involving garment production—from the plant fiber crop to the final production of a fabric and fashion design—it all needs to be in accordance with healthy, positive vibrations similar to the positive frequency and rhythm of the heart.

Take music, for instance. Music that goes against the resonance of the heart carries a negative frequency, a low vibration. In a study, they measured the frequency of specific music types. They either resonated or did not resonate with the heart based on their positive or negative frequency. The classical music genre yields the most positive frequencies. Traced back to its roots, instrumental music has ancient origins. Listening to the works of classical musicians can activate and upgrade human DNA, and support heart health at the cellular level. This is because of the positive frequencies and vibrations within the music.

According to geneticist Susumu Ohno, "The energy of the heart right down to the DNA is musical and rhythmic in nature. It cannot stop beating or else death typically occurs." At the Beckman Research Institute of the City of Hope in Duarte, California, Ohno translated four nucleotides from strands of DNA. Ohno compared and converted them to music. When this music was performed, listeners compared it to Bach, Brahms, and Chopin.

Music frequency in fashion

Civilization will advance when we incorporate more music and sound in fashion design. One way to incorporate new rhythms and frequencies of music in fashion is through the development of new knitwear machines that include new weaving techniques that imitate music patterns that are associated with positive frequencies.

Another way to incorporate music in fashion is with cymatic therapy. Cymatics is the study of sound and vibration. The cymascope, or cymatic device, is built of a metal plate connected to an oscillator. Sand is placed on the metal plate. When the oscillator is turned on, the sound frequencies vibrate the sand particles on the metal plate, and the sand is turned into geometric shapes that clearly have a visible, positive light frequency.

The oscillators produce a broad spectrum of sound frequencies. We can use these shapes and form them into fabrics and fashion designs. This will help upgrade and advance human DNA. We could also use cymatics in fashion by vibrating the threads and fabrics themselves with these sound frequencies. Numerous options to be developed are available.

Frequency of animal-derived fabric

The frequency of animal-based fashion products may be altered and manipulated negatively. Animal-derived fabrics and materials are primarily dead protein fibers. They are from either the skin of a dead animal, or animal hairs that are dead cells. The frequency of animal fiber is bound up with emotional states developed over time. Emotions both positive and negative are built up within the animal. These emotions can remain static within the skin, fur, and animal textiles. Animal fabrics can't neutralize human emotions like plant-based fabrics. Plant-based fabrics purify air and stagnant emotions. Animals are more like emotional sponges and their emotions can crystallize in parts of the animals' bodies. Sometimes, wearing leather accessories like purses or wallets is a way to connect with our own pain, because of the energy and emotions and memories that were painful that are still within a person, they align with the animal-based materials' frequencies that are made up of painful emotions.

Energetic frequency of plant-based fabric

Plant-based fabrics contain a high frequency, a "living" component. Plants break down in production, but the fabric is not "dead." Plant-derived fabrics are medicinal material, making them life-giving. Take dried herbs and spices, for instance. They may presumably be considered "dead," but when taken internally, in cooking or supplementation, they contain numerous nutrients and medicinal properties.

When they're dried, their frequency is high and their medicinal properties are intact, and there is still an inherent amount of healing properties within them. Similarly, there is no dead vibration after the plant fiber is converted to fabric. As the material is broken down into plant-based fabrics, its living essence remains intact.

Plant-based fabrics are made from sun, water, and soil, all of which vibrate naturally. Humans need sun, water, and soil to survive. Wearing plant-based fabrics is a direct route to wearing the Earth and Universe's vibration. There are ways of creating alchemy through the fabric development process which can alter fabric positively.

Something to consider is the point of integration between positive and negative which is the frequency of the sun, 126.22 Hz. There's something about the sun's frequency which transcends and does not neutralize vibration. This can symbolize the ratio of cellulose, being mostly made of half oxygen and half carbon. These two elements do not neutralize energy, yet transcend energy at a point of integration.

The frequency of linen

Dr. Otto Heinrich Warburg, a twentieth-century German doctor and scientist, made a very significant discovery. He found that linen holds a positive, high frequency at the atomic level. Research indicates that the frequency of linen is measured at 5,000 angstroms compared with synthetic, petroleum-derived fabrics positioned at a negative frequency. Because of its high frequency, linen naturally increases the life-force of the human body.

Bear in mind, we can't rule out the benefits of other fabrics if they are not measured at the same "high" frequency as linen because there are different ways of measuring the different forms of frequencies for their health factors, and they need to be more developed and considered. Each plant has a frequency with considerable advanced properties that are expressed differently. Each plant fiber produces their own, unique health benefits.

It has been scientifically proven that wool and linen—the energetic frequency of these two fibers—when combined and worn together collapse the energetic field. Linen combined with wool neutralizes the electrical field, creating a stuck and stagnant energy field. The difference is noticeable but it may be hard to detect for many people. Of course, though, being warm is more important. Wool can be a very important fabric to keep people warm when other fabrics are not an option.

As is suggested in the Book of Moses, also known as the Torah and Pentateuch, linen acts as an antenna to attract energy, nature's life-force, and divine consciousness. In a Japanese study, researchers dressed hospital beds with bedclothes made of linen fabric. Over time, they found no bedsores on patients compared with generic sheets that induced bedsores.

Dr. Phillip Callahan, a researcher and physician, found, when pure linen was placed over a wound or painful injury, it greatly accelerated the healing process. Additionally, at the electrical, cellular level, flax cells are highly complementary with human cells. Linen-based, internal sutures are used in the medical industry, because human cells are capable of completely dissolving flax cells.

Protecting and keeping the human aura healthy with fashion

The aura, or human energy field, consists of multiple layers of etheric energy. It is a halo within and around the body expanding outward at a radius of several feet. Some say the aura is a link to divine consciousness. Auras are seen depicted in fine-art paintings of various holy saints and spiritual figures. The aura can be seen from Kirlian photography (high-voltage electro photography), which is a photographic process that can detect and reveal a variety of different prismatic colors around humans and objects.

Healthy fashion directly cooperates with a human's auric/ energetic, electromagnetic field.

Clothing can assist in either strengthening or weakening a person's aura. As a person's vibration becomes higher, their aura becomes stronger. The electromagnetic energy of the body is like an antenna, it needs to be adjusted, balanced, and fueled. Clothing can be like a battery that charges the aura.

Clothing can work with the human aura as it transmits

and receives energy. Covering part of the aura in a variety of colored, plant-based fabrics will strengthen it and assist in clearing energy blockages. Many synthetic fabrics can suppress the aura, weakening and lessening its expansion. This decreases the aura's ability to clear negative energies within the body as well as it decreases the aura's ability to clear a person's external environment.

Fashion can protect the aura. Not only the fabrics of a garment, but its design can hinder or strengthen the aura: the protective energetic, etheric layer of the body. Fashion can also protect the meridians, chakras, and their magnetic forces. A garment's shape, color, fit, size, design, seams, proportion, pattern, material, and so on, are all important and need to be recognized and understood when using clothing as a tool to enhance and support the aura.

Fashion for protection: a natural shield of armor

Materials can be used as protective elements against new, past, or conditional environmental hazards. Electrical EMFs, electrical power plants, radioactive fumes, nuclear bomb leaks, carbon air pollution, chemical smog, virus epidemics, infection, nanotechnology, chemtrails, and foreign parasitic matter, visible or non-visible to the human eye, cannot be overlooked. Fashion can be used as a shield to protect the body, keeping it healthier and freer from these pollutants. Many people unconsciously adorn themselves with jewelry, accessories and clothing that specifically work to protect them.

Fashion found in sacred tombs

There were archeological finds from Europe, China, and the Middle East where fabrics, materials, and fashion remnants were discovered. Ancient Egyptians used fashion as a spiritual conductor and for protection. Mummies wrapped in various types of fabrics and protective materials to preserve the body were found inside the tombs in pyramid cell chambers. These materials can be further examined and utilized for the contemporary world, to help preserve the living body too, and used for their anti-aging effects.

These fabric wrapping techniques were not only used to preserve a dead body. Wrapping the mummy was a part of a ritual, and it would supposedly initiate a healthy afterlife. Many techniques that the ancients used to preserve mummies can serve not only the afterlife but also a living body in order to attain mystical and scientific-based health effects.

Cellulose-based plant fibers and their natural protective properties

Cellulose is the most abundant organic compound found on Earth. Major sources of cellulose fibers are cotton, linen, hemp, ramie, nettle, and lyocell. Cellulose fibers support the wearer because of the protective cell walls found in plants. A plant's cell walls support the plant structurally and support the body too.

Humans function well when eating fibrous, cellulose foods, as they act as a natural cleansing agent to purify the intestines and rid the body of disease. Cellulose-based fabrics slough off impurities on the skin, similar to the way cellulose fiber food sloughs off debris in the intestines. Their breathability property allows dead skin cells to naturally move away from the skin without re-imbedding or clinging to the skin.

There are natural protective functions of a plant's cell walls, like their geometrical structure that maintains its shape, supporting and strengthening plants. Additionally, cell walls in plants resist water pressure, withstand internal pressure, control cell growth, and regulate its metabolic processes. These same functions support the performance of plant-based fabrics.

Plant fiber cellulose has a semi-permeable property, allowing certain substances to diffuse through fabric while keeping other substances out. In a plant, this barrier prevents a viral attack. Plant fibers have antibacterial, anti-fungicidal, and bug-resistant properties, but still allow water, air, and other natural elements to pass through, supporting both the fabric and the body.

The cell walls of cellulose fiber retain moisture needed to support thermoregulation, a property necessary in fabrics to keep the body hydrated and pH-balanced, as the body is already made of 50–75% water. Cellulose contains many small holes within its crystalline-like structure. It's like the tubular structure of a flower stem with its many fibrous, spongy layers of holes absorbing moisture and nutrients. Cellulose-based fiber provides natural skin hydration. This additional moisture barrier for the body keeps one feeling fresher and keeps skin better moisturized.

The body's natural perspiration mechanism releases toxins. Cellulose-based fabrics do not suppress sweat as they act as an agent for healthy, natural perspiration. Plant stems and leaves bleed water throughout the entire outer structure, maintaining moisture balance. Overall, this is another reason why we should be wearing plant-based fashion.

Chapter 4

Healthy Fashion for the Spirit Body

Spiritual fashion is healthy fashion

The act and ritual of dressing is a prayer, a salutation, a poem, a movement, and creates an energetic shield of protection. It's a concentrated expression of union with self. It is an acknowledgement of the integrity of being, and instills a course of divine action. Clothing can be a tool to attract more divinity, when we wear the spirit of the Universe and divine consciousness.

There's a living consciousness within fabric that remains and does not die until disintegration. Spiritual consciousness within fabric and design is a valuable resource and refuge. Fashion can be used to work for oneself. As the great spiritual awakening occurs, fashion is becoming a tool for healing, right down to the activation of human DNA. It works to preserve, to rejuvenate, to prosper a person in the moment, and to achieve mind/body healing.

Fashion as a spiritual conduit cannot be overlooked. Spiritually connecting with fashion removes the error of superficially disconnecting with it. Fashion can enable a person to delve into heightened states of awareness. This creative, receptive, flow-like occurrence makes people feel more aware, and more comfortable in their own skin. This is a spiritual fashion intervention, an endeavor that offers more open-mindedness towards human existence. It is a part of a person's experience made of reflection in a soulful way.

No one is alone when they're dressed in clothing that's in union with their own soul. We are in constant connection with fabric, the "second skin." We really can have a relationship with our wardrobe, and it's a reflection of our relationship to ourselves, a reflection of our spirit. The relationship we have with fashion is not just a material pursuit. Clothing is energy, a life-force, and a source of divinity. It is not always about what clothing we attract. There will always be pieces of clothing in our wardrobe influenced by one's path, beliefs, experiences, and personal representation of self.

Spiritual fashion is not religious

Spiritual fashion merges with one's own personal faith. Spirituality is faith rooted from a human existing on purpose. Research studies prove that a spiritually driven life, one found through faith or a higher, divine power, creates a healthier mind and body.

The kind of spirituality I am referring to is in support of the growth of a person's spirit and soul through fashion. The term "spirituality," as it is expressed in this book, is universal. Most all forms of sacred religions are included, provided that they don't threaten humans or the Earth. Spiritual fashion does not reference specific religions unless they're connected to ancient and traditional lineages, before religion became an act of segregation.

Spiritual fashion illustrates an all-universal message that accepts all faith bases, yet excludes anything of evil or of satanic origin. Evil or negative fashion is void of spirit. A spiritless existence creates disconnection. This disconnection creates more strain and challenge for a person.

Disconnected, spiritless fashion is made of synthetic, artificial materials that don't feed the soul. It's challenging for many synthetic fabrics to hold spiritual consciousness due to their chemical composition. The fusion of toxic chemicals combined can disrupt spiritual consciousness. It performs and functions to the best of its ability, but it's not as spiritually aligned like natural plant-based fabrics are. Yet, there are synthetic-based fabrics and fashions that can be considered healthy, it's just not common.

It's not only about the fabric, but the design and fit of

garment. There are many plant-based garments that are negative too, simply because of the cut, design, or fit. For example, a natural linen garment that constricts the body. This goes against the body's need for natural movement, so, the spiritual consciousness of the plant fabric and garment diminishes. If it suppresses the breath, it's constricting life-force, and life-force is made up of divine consciousness. So, there are various factors that make a garment spiritual.

Fashion is denatured and spiritless when processed in an unclean, negative way. Through the administration of chemicals, its artificial structure, or its faulty design, they cannot be pure. They can't always be a vessel for divine consciousness when the fabrics and designs are disturbed. Yet, because spiritual consciousness is so vast, it has the ability to override many of these issues to a degree. For example, if a garment is made with synthetic fibers yet the design itself is ergonomic, and very comfortable. If people are comfortable then they are in a state and feeling of purity, and that feeling is divine.

Synthetic fabrics are not necessarily "evil," but many are "negative." There is a difference between pure and impure clothing. The Spiritual Science Research Foundation speaks about the spiritual effects of clothes. They explain that cotton, for instance, carries "sattvic" vibrations. Sattvic is an Indian Sanskrit term meaning healthy, balanced, and whole. They explain that sattvic, plant-based materials can supply energy to the body to achieve harmony. They also explain that synthetic fabrics, like polyester, are "tamasic" (toxic), and they can deplete the energy body.

The spiritual disconnect between humans and fashion is a serious threat. Intentionally or unintentionally, clothing can be anti-faith, evil-based, and in extreme cases act as a portal for satanic control or possession. Spirited fashion protects people from negative interference and possession. The toxic and evil threats disappear when fashion is merged with a person's soulful, spirited journey backed up by a positive force.

We can interpret a person's soul by their way of dress. There is a well-known saying: "Don't let yourself be eye candy, be soul food." Fashion depicted as eye candy is soulless, unpleasant, artificial, superficial, neither grounded nor balanced. Soulful fashion expresses a person's spiritual essence, conveying a spiritual type of awareness. At its strongest, spirit-filled fashion interferes with, and removes, the spiritless fashion properties that attempt to fracture, hinder, or lose a soul-expressed identity. Spiritless fashion can weaken the soul/spirit, and can make us feel vulnerable.

There is no doubt about how important it is to develop the role and relationship between fashion, humans, and spirit combined. Fashion is a pattern, a frequency, an uninterrupted sequence that gives off a specific rhythm. When this frequency is tapped, an unseen force like divine consciousness may not be easily recognizable, but it's there. We need this creative, divine, spiritual expression in fashion.

Fashion bound by nature, with all its vibrancy and beauty, is spirited fashion. Healthy, spirited fashion is made of plants and elements found in nature that are not toxic to the body. Incorporating elements of nature connects us with life's essence.

Plants are highly evolved forms of spiritual intelligence. All plants have a spirit. Nature is spirit-filled. Wearing nature gets people closer to their own inner spirituality. Materials like crystals, gems, and botanical dyes are beautiful and spiritually uplifting. When fashion is influenced by nature, we engage with the life-force of the physical body congruent with life-force of the physical earth.

Fashion as a navigational tool

Not only is fashion a creative expression, it's in constant

communication with the direct self. The human/fashion relationship forms a roadmap throughout a person's journey. Clothing then becomes a navigational tool, like a compass, to lead, direct, and guide us. It is like a prayer that is being called out for Great Spirit or for the Universe to hear. Clothing can actually lead us to new experiences and opportunities. The valuable direction that clothing gives us is not always acknowledged but it's consciously or unconsciously felt.

Everyone develops themselves through their own way of dress, no matter what kind of fashions they wear, or how they participate in fashion. It is a ritualistic creative process, to dress each day. When we embrace the connection that we have with fashion, it is sustaining the recognition of it being a sacred act.

There's no question that having a healthy wardrobe involves forming a sustaining relationship with dress. It's a soul-defining practice and initiates spiritual union with self, community, and the environment. Clothing offers stories that enhance life. Rather than clothing being used just as a catalyst, clothing plays a role, acting as an initiator in creating experiences.

There is a deeper, synchronistic purpose behind fashion design that interacts with a person's human experience. Synchronicities that come about from fashion may be proof that it can be a catalyst for divine intervention. Observed patterns of color, texture, shape, and designs create a force field of synchronistic connectivity. The patterns found in fashion, both worn and seen, form like a poem or a puzzle of life's interconnectedness, yet they are not all merely visible color or design combinations. There's significance behind patterns just like the patterns found in sacred geometry. Patterns in dress are something to be conscious of. They can attract specific, positive rhythms to one's being.

Galactic-inspired fashion

Galactic-inspired fashion is spiritual fashion. It's a new, multidimensional way of being and appearing. Clothing can be a perfect foundation to enable galactic communication for deeper mind expansion, and help connect people with the Universe's cosmic, energy currents. This empowered clothing type, "galactic fashion," eliminates destructive fashion misaligned with the Universe's natural rhythms.

Galactic fashion makes spiritual ascension more and more possible, because it's a metaphysical tool and healing modality. This is an important part of fashion's evolution: to go beyond taking inspiration from the surface of the Earth, and take inspiration from the universe, or multiverse. We are respecting the fashion industry, and we are respecting our own fashion intelligence when we embrace this new fashion idea. In order to introduce new fashion ideas that communicate beyond the typical style genres, we have to embrace our instinctual desire for mind expansion. When the mind is open, it is open to new fashion ideas.

This idea of galactic fashion transpired through my interest in space, the supernatural, and from the idea of creating fashion, designed to ascend the body, mind, and spirit. Galactic fashion is a pertinent tool for human growth. It introduces cosmic elements that are aligned with Earth's divine perfection. When this type of apparel is worn, the energy body is fueled.

Fortunately, clothing can be used as a channel to connect humans with other multidimensional universes. The human race on planet Earth has ancestral ties with aliens on other planets in the universe. We don't have complete proof that there is life on other planets, but there is a lot of evidence that aliens exist. If we exist, it is most likely possible that other beings exist on other planets.

It is hard to imagine alien life because it's not something right in front of us or in pictures for us to see. As time passes,

I believe the planetary ascension activity will advance the human race to the point where we will have full capability to visualize and interpret our multidimensional universe, and experience it to greater depths. For example, astral travel, meditation, and the third eye, are a few ways to access parallel universes.

There's a new need to develop supernatural, galactic fashion. In order for that to happen we need to perceive the idea that Earth is not just "earthy," it's a "supernatural" phenomenon. Earth is a planet just like the other planets in the galaxy, and when we think about other planets, they often appear as way more space-age and alien-like. We are "earthlings" in the grand scheme of things, so this planet needs to claim its own space-age and alien-like aspects, and not appear as separate from the galactic picture.

Planet Earth is not earthy at all, we have just been programmed to see it that way. Earth, the forest and its natural elements can be perceived as modern. Nature has supernatural capabilities, not all are recognized. The future of fashion is galactic, and universal.

To treat clothing as only an "earthy" embodiment does not give fashion enough substance and new fashion potential. Fashion design that is celestial, futuristic, space-age, with influences of other style genres to pare it down so they don't look like costumes, will help support the new, upcoming trend of galactic-inspired fashion. Additionally, marketing plant-based fabrics and plant-based dyes, not as earthy, yet as supernatural and futuristic, and also marketing fashion design that goes beyond the planet Earth and is inspired by new dimensions, this will help create more promise towards modern fashion.

Clothing can be used as a vehicle, a form of transport to other worlds known or unknown, and can help initiate multidimensional states of consciousness for ultimate wellbeing. The galaxy plays a critical part in existence. Tapping into the sun, moon, stars, planets, and galaxy allows a universal interconnection of healing to occur. Black holes, meteorites, spiral galaxies, hypervelocity stars, and other things in outer space can be used to influence fashion design for the benefit of creating supernatural fashion. This can be achieved in the color, fabric, design, construction, pattern, cut and silhouette of a fashion design.

Galactic light codes in fashion

One way to make fashion a metaphysical, spiritual tool and healing modality is adding galactic light codes to apparel and accessories. Galactic codes are energetic symbols that convey cosmic patterns, sacred geometry, sound, and frequency. They transmit a positive energy and light frequency. Galactic codes are a kind of language that offers us an opportunity to open up to a new form of "galactic fashion communication." Galactic codes support the great spiritual awakening, and planetary ascension.

Some call galactic codes a "starseed" light language. Starseeds are individuals who believe they may have originated from another world, dimension, or planet. Galactic codes are for everyone, whether a person thinks they are a starseed or not. They form a language within the depths and layers of their design and symbol. This language can move people into cosmic realms, as it disperses knowledge that is ancient and rooted from the entire Universe.

Galactic light codes are often found in sacred geometry and in the hieroglyphics of Ancient Egypt. Galactic codes, when activated, become light portals to transcend energy. When light codes connect with a human's spirit body, the frequency is transferred. The healing properties of galactic light codes are similar to energy healing and crystal therapy. They transmute negativity, block bad energy, and activate and repair DNA to advance human consciousness.

Galactic light codes contain octaves of rhythm and movement similar to the musical tones that come from a musical instrument. These codes are definitely musical by nature. They all contain an encoded pattern, and they can come from geometric shapes like holograms, pyramids, merkaba crystal grids, and vortexes.

Many existing textile patterns and prints could be made more useful if they were purposefully made as a light code, to produce a positive energy transmission. A galactic symbol or print on a garment can be a visual meditation that alters consciousness. Design elements such as symbol, pattern, movement of a silhouette, shape, texture, and physical dimension can help the formation of new light-code transmissions for the wearer and viewer.

When wearing or viewing textile prints, many of them naturally add more depth in emotion, human thinking, and perception. Symbols can be profound for therapeutic use, however simple or in-depth they look. Fashion designs that have textile printed light code patterns onto the fabric, or they are woven or knitted into the fabric, they are a way to open up the mind.

The redundancy of some basic prints like plaid, polka dots, and stripes can exhaust the mind and the immune system, due to their bare, commercial-like, generic look. There's definitely a place and time for stripes, polka dots, and checks, yet sometimes these types of prints can become kind of dull and mind-numbing with not enough depth and feeling. At times, basic prints provide flow and interest. They can be artistic and inspiring when a look is styled successfully. Yet many basic prints can only do so much for a person. It really depends on the intention and the design of a print/pattern and how it is worn; this is what brings a pattern to life.

How does one go about detecting galactic light codes in

fashion? Light codes are common in artwork, not as much in fashion. Whether light codes are visually recognized and felt or not, there is a subconscious energy transfer that occurs. Light code apparel will gradually become more detectable when it becomes more in trend. Depending on a person's experience, some people react much more sensitively than others to the observation and feeling of light codes. It's like having the gift of being an energy worker; not everyone has the innate ability to feel and sense energy, but energy workers do. However, light codes are not only for people that can see or sense them.

People that are drawn to notice light codes may be practicing spirituality or metaphysical subjects attentively, or they may have the gift of intuition. Yet some codes are truly not visible. Some are seen and others are hidden. It is a person's unconscious working with the light codes. Light codes can be open for interpretation as well. They are personal to each individual. Their powers work by the beholder's own perception and experience as well. Light codes are not always up to visual interpretation, however.

Galactic-inspired fashion helps the environment

Wearing galactic apparel can offer benefits to a wearer's surrounding environments and spaces. How does this work? Take a crystal, for example. Crystals are placed on the ley lines of sacred areas around the world. The concept of ley lines was developed by Alfred Watkins. These are invisible, electromagnetic paths that connect each sacred site from all around the world, together. They are a part of the Earth's electric grid. When crystals are placed near or around these energy vortexes and ley lines, the crystal's healing properties and healing powers are heightened. These crystals then act as antennas, and as concentrated force fields of light contributing to the planet's ascension. When placed in those specific locations, they also broadcast outward.

So, say a garment is made up of these crystals. When a person wears a crystal-based garment, and visits sacred areas in their location, these crystals and the person's energy body can become more activated as they become connected to the ley lines of the planet. The crystals can then disperse positive energy around the wearer and their environment.

Celestial, galactic apparel, made with crystals for example, can clear energy blockages in and around an area that is low vibration or polluted. Our clothing, if it's properly designed to do so, can amplify positive energy and divine consciousness, and purify these polluted areas, just by the fabrics and fashion designs merged with a human's energy and spirit body.

Purifying the negative energy in polluted areas can also occur with the help of the person's intention through prayer, mantra, or by active meditation. Galactic apparel can be used as a healing tool to heal, recover, and purify a person's surroundings, wherever they may be. These fashion designs will work to draw out impurities within the body, and balance and dismantle blocked energy issues within a concentrated area or larger radius of land. This is the future of galactic fashion.

Prismatic fashion

Prismatic, holographic fashion has healing powers rooted from ancient times. Opalescent, iridescent, prism, rainbow-like apparel is spiritual fashion. Rainbows symbolize the celebration of life. They can boost mood and positivity levels. The Incans believed that rainbow colors are a divine manifestation of sun and rain. The rainbow symbolizes a connection between heaven and Earth. When merging feminine and masculine qualities together, the prism encompasses the whole of the yin and yang energy of a person's spirit.

The rainbow is the most widely used LGBT symbol in the world. The rainbow flag was invented by Gilbert Baker in

1978, for the Gay Freedom Pride parade. The issue with this is, it takes away some of the magic of what a rainbow truly represents, a symbol of "all of life." If it is associated with only a person's sexual orientation, this is a form of suppressing the rainbow. This is narrowing and limiting the use of the rainbow in fashion. Everyone should be able to be entitled to have a spiritual, magical association with the rainbow colors. Using rainbow colors in the form of the prism diffuses the idea that rainbows represent LGBT pride only. There needs to be more fashion designs that can transmute the rainbow symbol so it can symbolize all.

A full spectrum of visible light travels through the prism, containing healing wavelengths of the electromagnetic spectrum. It is also understood that the color rays of a prism are spiritual forces that flow from white light. The prism creates pure light separated into various wavelengths that are said to be individual aspects of God. Wearing prismatic, holographic textiles can enhance and produce more crystalline prism energy within the body and human aura. This supports kundalini activation. Enhancing, protecting, and cultivating a rainbow aura increases health.

Examples of prismatic fashion are fabrics that are sparkling, effervescent, shimmering, lustrous fabrics. Shimmer fabrics that glisten like water reflecting the sun are shields of armor, creating a warrior-like barrier. Prismatic fashion enhances the body, adorning it to protect spirit within, and upon Earth.

Sacred holy symbols worn

Holy symbols in fashion yield power. They bless the wearer and onlooker. They can be integrated into a garment as a textile print, embroidery, weave or as a jewelry accessory. Many cultures and people around the world place significance on the use of symbols being decoratively displayed on clothing, claiming they hold spiritual purposes.

Ceremonial clothing is spiritual fashion. They have a certain spiritually commanding power. It's not limited to just robes or priestly garments. Trend-driven designs influenced by ceremonial dress can be made to reflect their spiritual strength and power. The sacredness of ceremonial clothing prompts a deeper sense of connection to life, enforcing a sense of self-empowerment. These "holy" garments can attract divine consciousness and simultaneously repel evil, or negative consciousness.

Here are a few examples of sacred, spiritual attire that hold ancient lineage and are still being represented today:

The ankh symbol: The ankh is a very powerful ancient symbol representing life and eternal existence. Used as a healing tool, it can transmit light energy. The ankh symbol is said to open the door to the afterlife and other dimensions. There has also been mention of it being the original Holy Cross.

The robe: The robe holds power. Beginning in ancient times it was worn prominently in religious sectors of society. Monks, swamis, rabbis, priests/priestesses, Ascended Masters, angels, they all wear a robe in some form of style. The robe symbolizes the spiritual kingdom. Nothing can replicate its spiritual power, and the same can be said for other sacred garments, as well. There are different, stylish renditions of the robe. Design alterations and adaptations to the robe silhouette can be integrated into fashion as a modern-day, "holy" fashion trend.

The orange robe: Indian swamis and Buddhist monks wear orange-colored robes primarily. The orange color symbolizes the sunlight that casts out and expels darkness. When you observe a monk or a swami's robe, without a doubt there is a visible, holy sentiment attached to it, an expression of holy power. The robe, when worn, blesses the passerby and blesses the wearer. This kind of power is sacred, and comes from a higher consciousness.

The seamless tunic of Jesus: The day Jesus was crucified, his robe was stripped and taken from him. His seamless tunic/robe was unable to tear or be ripped apart. When he was still living, people discovered if they touched Jesus' garment they were immediately cured. There are testimonies of this occurrence stated in the Bible. This is a testament to the power of cloth; that divine consciousness can work through the fabrics that are laid upon a human body. The cloth may also become a living embodiment of the person's essence and spirit.

The robe of the ephod, worn by the high priest of Israel: The robe of the ephod was worn before the Lord so that the high priest would be blessed to continue living. This garment is described as being full of symbolism and was used for divination purposes. The ephod robe has a bell attached to it, to banish all evil. It was made with a breastplate of 12 gemstones resting over the heart and chest for protection.

Gold, purple, blue, scarlet, and white are its main colors. These colors were used to convey spiritual significance and divine messages. Its gold thread symbolizes divine righteousness. Blue means "Jesus is All God." God made the sky blue to represent the glory of his Son who is "All blue." Purple symbolizes the color of royalty and intuitive divinity. Lastly, red, meaning red-blooded man, symbolizes the blood Jesus shed. The white linen tunic worn underneath the robe symbolizes purity and righteousness.

Prayer shawl: Prayer shawls honor the soul. The prayer shawl is originally known as the *tallit* in Hebrew. Biblically, it is known as a visible symbol of the word of God. It is described as: "A commanded blessing given by God." The tassels, or *tzit tzitot*, were a later addition. The Lord spoke to Moses and told him to add tassels at the corners of the shawl, with a blue thread in remembrance of the commandments of the Torah. The term *tzit tzitot* is translated as "wings to flee and get away." The blue thread is called *shamash*, "helper," and the blue color symbolizes heaven and royalty.

The weaving of the *tallit* garment is produced on a spiritual level. This makes the garment even more holy, protective, healing, and a blessing to wear. The Jewish people created a specific, spiritual, tassel wrapping method to produce the tassels representing Hebrew letters which indicate the name of God: YHVH, meaning "I Am That I Am." Thus, the making of the garment is akin to a spiritual ceremony or ritual. The spiritual command of the entire tassel arrangement is God saying: "I Am your healer, your provision. I Am because I Am."

The dress of the Ascended Masters

The Ascended Masters are spiritual figures, a group of spiritually enlightened beings that were once humans. They are of good nature and dress in a holy way. They have a masterly ability and resemble that of high priests and priestesses. They use fashion not only for their own benefit, but also to invoke special, supernatural powers. Clothing for them is used as an instrument for divine manifestation and for spiritual activation to occur.

The robe is the most popular silhouette and a consistent style staple in the attire of most spiritual figures. This garment can be adapted and updated to fit a person's needs and aesthetic taste. Because their dress is influential and inspirational, as most costume or holy attire is, it is important to modernize and integrate their way of dress into our current wardrobes, because people will be turned off if it appears too costume-like.

This is in order to make fashion an instrument for supernatural powers to occur. You don't need a garment to activate spiritual consciousness or supernatural powers within, but like any tool or healing modality, they are a catalyst for ultimate healing and spiritual ascension.

Fashion and spiritual figures as forms of inspiration: Ascended Masters and their soul colors

The Ascended Masters are believed to be people who have gone through a series of initiations and spiritual transformation which eventually brought them to a point where they achieved enlightenment. They all have a certain mastery over a specific offering. They are both physical and non-physical, meaning they are multidimensional beings and do not always need to be in a physical body in order to survive and exist. They exist primarily in spiritual reality.

Each Ascended Master typically has a color that they work with. Colors do not only represent a mood or feeling, they can perform. This goes way beyond color symbolism, it's color performing.

Colors can hold power. The colors associated with the Ascended Masters are power sources of energy cultivated over time. Usually their signature soul color is the dominant color found in their aura.

A well-known Ascended Master, St. Germain, associated with the color purple, represents the violet flame. He wears a violet purple colored robe, and it activates the "violet flame." He is not merely associating with the color; he is a representation of the force of that color. His robe of violet purple creates a beam of violet light. His soul color, as represented in his robe, is also directed outward onto the onlooker, and it heals them. So, Ascended Masters are using their colored garments to help other people and the environment, not only themselves.

The violet flame is said to purify the soul. So, St. Germain's garment purifies the soul of people who see it. It also purifies the soul of the planet. So, instead of only the Ascended Master's mind and body being the "spiritual channel," the garment becomes the spiritual channel, too. Additionally, Ascended Masters can also be associated with more than one color.

We can use color as a source of power and as an energetic force that initiates and works as a portal/channel for divine healing to occur within oneself, and extend it throughout the Universe, like these Ascended Masters do. Additionally, in Buddhism or Eastern Indian religious traditions, orange and white colors are used as a testament to their level of spiritual .stature and commitment to their religious/spiritual path. Orange and white are part of their soul colors, and they become an embodiment of their spiritual power.

There are also "soul colors" associated with a person's own, individual, soul path. Soul colors can interchange and reflect the times, as well, during the course of a lifetime or of an eternal lifetime. We are meant to tap into colors to initiate a "spiritual essence" and "soul presence." Soul colors are lively, with luminescent, pearlescent, and iridescent properties. An individual can tap into colors associated with the numerous Ascended Masters for rapid healing and self-realization. This can lead to the discovery of the truth behind what colors can ultimately represent in fashion, and how they can be used in a divine way for health and wellbeing.

Ascended Masters and their multidimensional clothing

In the book, *The Magic Presence*, by Godfre Ray King (Guy Ballard), the author goes into great detail about the Ascended Masters' clothing. There are several things to consider. Their clothing and fashion materials activate consciousness, and unblock stuck energy or unwanted negativity. Their materials are divine in nature, and come from nature, and are for the greater good.

Crystals are an important feature displayed on an Ascended Master's ensemble. The adorned crystals are designed in geometric formations similar to the breastplate of the ephod robe, made with various gems. Crystals can be placed in certain areas of the body for their health properties. It is the way they are designed into a look to be used as a form of armor that is most important. Additionally, it is the way they are designed with other materials that ignite the gems and make the gems "activate."

An example of an Ascended Master's healing crystal design formation is the brilliance of a white crystal, shaped in a circle, with dozens of tiny white crystals surrounding the larger white crystal centerpiece. The crystals are embedded in a rose-gold or soft white-gold metal material that delicately wraps around the neck and hangs down onto the upper chest.

Other examples of Ascended Master clothing can be found and depicted in the artworks made and inspired by the I AM teachings. One artwork showcases an accessory cuff displayed on the wrist of an Ascended Master, who is made to appear like a spiritual warrior. The cuff is made of red rubies and sapphire blue stones resting on a plate in a very powerful, geometrical formation. These cuffs would be uncomfortable if they were to be reproduced and made of a heavy metal. The material choices would need to be changed and converted in order to produce an ergonomic design meant for the physical body to wear day to day. We would likely need to adapt the Ascended Masters' fashion designs depicted in the I AM channeled paintings so that they perform the same way, but are made to suit the body comfortably.

We can utilize jewelry, crystals, and accessory designs as a form of protection. They can also perform as an antenna, as crystals and minerals tend to broadcast and enhance the electromagnetic energy of ley lines and the human energy body. The ley lines work as a grid-like energy body for the planet that contributes to its planetary awakening and activation. Our clothing can be utilized in this way; as vehicles, channels, portals, and as an antenna. They also grant us more accessibility to the ley line energies that support us. There are vortexes all over the planet, connected to the photon belt, that harness and harbor the energies that are broadcast on Earth and out into the Universe.

The ley line energies bring humans closer to enlightenment because our energy is purified and enhanced by them. As the energies and vibrations rise, we can no longer be in a state of human suffering and negativity due to the activation and alignment of the Universe. The Earth is moving into its New Age, and we are at a time when supernatural occurrences will soon occur naturally. This is when our clothing will no longer be viewed from a lower perspective but from a higher, much more multidimensional one.

The fabrics described in *Magic Presence* are captivating. Their lucid, living, and glistening-like fabrics give off a flowing, liquid effect. This is not a case of imagination or fantasy, as it does sound like this material would be impossible to reproduce in real life; but this material can be achieved when working with energy and materials down to their cellular and molecular level. It is possible to build healthy fabrics that are luminescent.

It will take the correct practice in working with new and old materials, and creating fabrics that are inspired and designed with materials like plant-based glitters, and crystals that are neon and opalescent. This will not only activate higher thinking and support the body; it will also help the passerby on the receiving end.

Utilizing the properties of materials that not only protect the wearer, but move the mind into a state of purity and awareness, is part of this new method of fashion for health.

Take seaweed, for instance. This is an example of a material we can use to make fabric feel and look lucid, naturally. The texture and feeling of seaweed, the liquid-like movement in its still form, is a therapeutic quality. There is something quite magical and profound about seaweed that goes beyond the actual material. This quality can be utilized in fashion, to bring us into a state of relaxation, from its multidimensional state.

The texture, shape, or appearance of seaweed can purposefully be kept as part of a seaweed-based fabric's design through technological improvements. The seaweed plant itself could be the main source of material in the fabric. This is really about gravitating towards materials that are transcendent. Observing and wearing the liquid-like texture of seaweed promotes an effect of movement while being still. This can be used as a form of active meditation and to be used to help achieve enlightenment for the mind, body, and soul. This fluidity property in a fabric's surface appearance and texture gives health benefits, and can be fulfilled via various design elements and techniques.

PART 2

UNHEALTHY FASHION

Chapter 5

Unhealthy Fabrics

Fashion gone rogue

Part 2, "Unhealthy Fashion," is not included to promote fear or introduce more challenges than is already manageable. One large concern, however, is that we have relied on synthetic polyester, nylon, and acrylic for some time now. There are evident repercussions from them that come in the form of illness. I don't make claims that synthetic fabrics are toxic to the point where they are lethal or highly damaging. I believe they are disruptive to varying degrees, they can weaken the mind/body, and be a contributing factor to disease and suffering.

There are many examples of cases where they can become, or already are creating a health issue, but the body can handle some of the most severe outcomes caused by the use of some of the most severe, harsh, toxic materials of fabrics. Most importantly, I believe Great Spirit is in control over the situation. The textile and apparel industry are ready to work out the negative interference for Earth and its inhabitants.

There is no reason to burden or put blame on anyone wearing or producing unhealthy apparel, because we are all susceptible to it unconditionally. It's extremely challenging to get away from synthetic fabrics, especially in colder climate regions. For those that don't care to shop online, or can't, they get what's available in their local clothing shops. Some of us need that connection of trying a garment on before we decide to purchase it.

So, what is most available in stores and online shopping sites for cold-weather apparel is made of synthetic fabric, or cotton/poly blended fabric, unless it's wool or animal skin/fur. Many people can't tolerate the prickle and itch factor of wool. Until we improve our plant-based fabric developments, and increase their production, most synthetic coats and jackets are fine to wear if they're loose-fitting and ergonomic. Some synthetic apparel is made in such an ergonomic way that it can feel and look healthy. Everything is in transition.

Worldwide production of synthetic fabric totals 65% of all textiles annually. Cotton is at 21% production, an estimated 94% of which is genetically modified. Rayon viscose production totals 8%. Rayon viscose is artificial, because it's a chemical-converted fabric. Due to its chemical-based composition it can be categorized as semi-synthetic. Only 5% of textile production comprises plant-based fabrics, such as linen and hemp. Around 1% of textile production is wool. When the production of polyester, nylon, acrylic, and viscose rayon are combined, they make a total of 73% synthetic textile apparel production.

In 1980, the polyester demand produced globally was at 5.2 million tons. In 2000, polyester increased to 19.2 million tons. In 2014, polyester had increased to about 46.1 million tons. The increase is evident to us all. By 2025, it is said the textile industry will be 95% synthetic-based. I don't believe the projected percentage will hold true for the future; however, if there are no new plant-based fashion developments, they won't increase in demand, and changes won't occur.

The history of Monsanto and DuPont's synthetic fabrics

Monsanto, originally named Monsanto Chemical Company, and recently acquired by Bayer, they were one of the top initiators and producers of synthetic fabric production, beginning in the 1930s during the industrial boom. It is challenging to detect which chemical companies Monsanto owned, as they have acquired many companies under other company names. Their company, Solutia Inc., which had been acquired by Eastman Chemical Company, was once, and still is, one of the largest nylon manufacturers in America. Petroleum-based nylon is one of the most toxic fabrics available. Studies reveal that wearing nylon can lead to negative symptoms such as skin issues, allergies, dizziness, and more.

The Monsanto Company was a top nylon manufacturer. Cerex Advanced Fabrics was founded by Monsanto Company in 1996 and it is still operating. Cerex Advanced Fabrics Inc. is just what they say they are: "The world leader in the manufacturing and sales of spun-bond nylon and non-woven fabrics." Monsanto also branded an acrylic fabric, naming it Acrilan. Acrylic fabric is one of the most lethal of them all in regard to its carcinogenic property. One of their original company advertisements states: "For contemporary elegance, nothing beats wool, except Acrilan."

The first large-scale productions of PVC (poly-vinyl chloride) were made by Monsanto, Dow, and Shell Co. Phosgene is found in PVC during thermal decomposition. Gas-related fatalities from phosgene and diphosgene reached 85% in the First World War. PVC is currently banned for use in water pipes. Studies have shown the test experiments of PVC against animals have resulted in cancer, liver damage, growth defects, and immune system damage.

In 1929, Monsanto was the sole producer of PCBs, which were finally banned in 1979. However, PCBs in textile dyes are still showing up everywhere. A study by Rutgers University tested 16 yellow-dyed garments for PCB residue from a mass retailer. All 16 garments contained PCB-11. PCB-11 is an unregulated chemical, because its toxins are considered an "unintentional by-product." Exposure to PCBs can result in a slew of health problems.

Monsanto has not only affected the food industry with genetically modified foods, but they have also genetically modified fabrics too. Recently acquired by Bayer, Monsanto was the largest biotech company in the world and was the creator of genetically modified cotton. Chemical companies, predominantly Monsanto, were mass suppliers of artificial, genetically modified Bt cotton. Genetically engineering plants is an epidemic that artificially alters and transmutes the gene/ DNA of the plant.

DuPont is an American chemical company. They are the second-largest producer of chemicals in the world, and the fifth largest company in biotech. DuPont created several of the top toxic, synthetic fabrics: polyester, nylon, and acrylic.

DuPont also created Teflon in 1945, a water-repellent finishing treatment used on fabrics that is still being produced today. The sale of Teflon pots and pans is decreasing because their Teflon finish is poisoning people. Additionally, it takes 25 generations for PFOA, a chemical used in Teflon, to biodegrade, and they may have negative effects on the liver, immune, and endocrine systems. Exposure to these chemicals is a hazard and they should be discontinued.

The toxicity of synthetic fabrics

Chemists, producers and distributors of chemical products might argue that everything is potentially natural, even a chemical. Everything essentially can be called a chemical. However, not all natural substances are healthy to begin with and can be poisonous to the body. Many artificial ingredients do not resemble, or are not complementary to the natural elements of the human body or elements found in nature. Chemicals are altered and engineered to such a degree that they become toxic, unnatural synthetic substances, and poisonous due to their chemical composition and structure.

Not all chemicals are bad. For example, many vitamins are synthetic and manmade. They are not natural, but they are beneficial and healthy for the body. Like synthetic vitamins, many manmade chemicals in textiles are healthy and non-toxic. What matters most is further examination of the use of these natural or manmade chemicals, and whether they are healthy or harmful to the body.

We can continue producing fabrics made with chemicals, but they need to be made with non-toxic chemicals, or made with plant-based chemicals. There is no need, though, to continue wearing synthetic materials with such a large load of chemicals when we can easily switch to plant-based fabrics, made with fewer chemicals.

There are 84,000 chemicals used in products with only 1% tested for safety. If apparel items are selling on the sales floor, people can assume it's safe to wear. This is not the case. Treated, synthetic fabrics in the industry are made with over 8,000 different chemicals, and they are not all safe. Studies reveal a host of harmful chemicals have been found in the bloodstream from wearing fabrics with chemicals.

According to the US Environmental Protection Agency (EPA), polyester, dicarboxylic acid, alcohol ethane, propane, esters of dihydric alcohol, and terephthalic acid ingredients used in synthetic fabrics may induce cancer. Some synthetic garments and accessories contain warning labels on their tags or stickered labels stating: "Warning, this product may cause cancer, birth defects, or reproductive harm." Additionally, when synthetic fabrics are burned, the smoke contains hydrogen cyanide. The EPA says this smoke may cause cancer. Additionally, it takes 30–40 years to decompose, emitting CO_2.

Synthetic fabrics are made from petroleum oil, coal, air, water, and numerous carcinogenic chemicals. They are composed mainly of 83–85% carbon. Carbon is acidic in nature. The body's elemental composition is mainly oxygen/hydrogen, so the predominantly carbon-based fabric can stress the body because it can be too acidic. Over-acidity is one of the main causes of disease.

The toxic chemical composition of synthetic fabrics, and their structure make them unbreathable. Most of them cannot be made breathable no matter how much technology is used. If a garment is loose-fitted, then the fabric won't be as much of a threat to the body, and is generally OK to wear. Skin has its own oxygen/breathing cycle, and when the skin's ability to breathe gets cut off by these synthetic materials, it will cause aging, discomfort, and block the body from its natural need to breathe through the skin.

Crude oil, polyester's main component, is comprised of decayed fossils of plants and animals that come as an oil derivative underneath the Earth's surface. Crude oil in its raw natural state is a thick, black sludge. As it is formed over time, it is naturally highly condensed and acidic. Oil spills are a serious threat to ocean life, so it's a wonder why it's used for apparel. For example, it threatens sea life; the oil destroys the insulating ability of the fur of sea otters. It also diminishes the water repellency of a bird's feathers. Sea animals can die from hypothermia, hypophagia, and suffocation when they are covered in petroleum oil.

We can consider that we are wearing the crude oil, topically, and can factor in how this can affect the body. Synthetic textiles are not the original form of crude oil, but based on what crude oil is made of, this should give us some idea of its ill-effects. Although these ill-effects may not be directly obvious from the appearance of synthetic apparel.

The tourist areas of Azerbaijan are known for their spas, which include Naftalan crude oil baths. Spa owners offer a bath of Naftalan crude oil as a spa treatment. There is much speculation as to whether this is actually healthy. A report was made on the side-effects and symptoms after getting out of the oil bath. They described feeling shaky, light-headed, and nervous.

Spa companies only allow their clients to bathe in the liquid petroleum for 10 minutes, and afterwards the oil is scrubbed off the body quite quickly. They say if a person were to stay in the bath any longer the oil could be detrimental to the heart and have a pernicious effect. As heart disease is the leading cause of death worldwide, synthetic fabrics may be playing a role. How? Crude oil-based fabrics that cover the body, especially when they fit tightly, create a block. The body can become stressed, and this puts a toll on human organs such as the heart.

We can also consider, we may be ingesting the release of microplastics from synthetic fabrics. Additionally, the synthetic nano-molecules in fabric finishing treatments can be absorbed through the skin. They could also be introduced into the bloodstream through this way. The chemicals and dyes of generic fabric can also be absorbed through the skin.

The Environmental Agency in Austria conducted a study of plastics found in human fecal matter. Several types of microplastics were found in the stool samples of eight participants. Up to nine microplastic types were found out of the ten that were tested. The most commonly found microplastics were polypropylene and polyethylene terephthalate. Polypropylene is a popular material in apparel, and polyethylene is the most common type of polyester used in the apparel industry.

Unhealthy fabrics and their negative side effects

The fabrics listed below are generally unhealthy. Synthetic fabrics should be used sparingly, and they would need to be very ergonomic and comfortable in order to be considered healthy fashion. There are synthetic garments that are healthy, simply from their design aesthetic. If the design makes a person happy, and it's comfortable to wear, it's healthy. Additionally, polyester and synthetic garments are not as harmful to wear in cold temperatures, because when it is cold, the body needs warmth, and the synthetic fabrics trap in the warmth.

Polyester is manmade, cheap to produce, and petroleum-based. When polyester garments are heated, from drying garments or by body heat, the chemicals embedded in the plastic fiber outgas. Additionally, it's hard for the skin to breathe when wearing polyester fabrics. They typically create a lack of movement, a non-ergonomic textile property.

The lint scattered all over the floors comes from fabrics, and they end up being inhaled through our nose and mouth. It's important to realize that tiny fragmented fiber particles can leach into the body. The particles potentially penetrate through the skin pores and orifices. Tiny pieces of plastic fibers, as well as chemicals from dyes and fabric treatments, are inhaled through the mouth and absorbed through the pores. They can eventually disperse into the bloodstream and the rest of the system.

Nylon is a petroleum-based fiber, containing toxic chemicals like cyclohexane and ammonia. Heated body temperature may potentially release these toxins. Nylon production creates nitrous oxide, a greenhouse gas that is 310 times more potent than carbon dioxide. Nylon does not easily decompose. It emits hazardous smoke when burned.

Acrylic is a petroleum-based fiber. It is the least breathable synthetic fiber. It often has a strong scent of toxic fumes emanating off of it. In 1979, the US Environmental Protection Agency (EPA) tested acrylic, and they made it known that the residual monomers in acrylic may be carcinogenic.

Rayon is made of plant cellulose; however, it is chemically processed and chemical-based. The cellulose pulp that is used to make rayon is converted into a fiber through heavy chemical processing. The conversion of cellulose by the chemical solvent makes it artificial. There's no way to distinguish what is part plant or part chemical after processing. It often has a soft feel that makes it appealing against the skin, yet the processing treatment uses several toxic chemicals like ammonia, acetone, carbon disulfide, sulfuric acid, chlorine, and caustic soda. The heavy use of chemical processing makes the fabric unhealthy to wear. Lyocell is a healthier option.

Sugar-derived synthetic fabrics Ingeo™, a bioplastic PLA fiber, is a corn-based, biosynthetic fabric, and falls into the category of genetically modified materials. Biobased synthetic fabrics are going to be an important trend, and they will be an important solution and substitute for petroleum-based synthetic fabrics, but not sugar-derived biobased fabrics. It is made to appear eco driven, yet the conversion, materials used, and processing methods make the product unhealthy to wear.

There is currently a surge in sugar-derived plastic fabrics becoming more popular in fashion apparel. These are viscose-processed, biobased materials made from food sources like corn, beets, and sugarcane. During the fabric manufacturing process, the corn is turned into an acid-producing corn sugar. Additionally, as in all viscose-made processing, heavy chemicals are used to break down and plasticize the fiber. Sugar-derived, biodegradable bioplastic is better off being used for packaging materials.

We go out of our way to cut sugar from our diet, yet wearing fabrics made from sugar invites the opportunity to "wear sugar." Sugar is acidic and a potential proponent of feeding cancer cells in the body. They do originate from plants, but sugar-based textiles are not a part of the plant-based fabrics list, because they promote illness. We can use other, healthier parts of these plants—for example, the corn's husk can be used as a textile (not the corn kernels)—for better use of them, and for their health properties.

Genetically modified fabrics An estimated 1 to 5 million cases of pesticide poisoning occur each year. There have been 220,000 reported deaths annually, with at least 1 million requiring hospitalization, from pesticide poisoning. 99% of these deaths occur in the developing world. More than 270,000 Indian cotton farmers have killed themselves since 1995. 95% of Indian cotton farms are using genetically modified cotton seeds and pesticides on their crops. Investigators have said there are various factors as to their recent suicidal death increase, but it's clear many are working on genetically modified cotton farms, so there is a connection.

Another problem with GMO crop farming: the genetically modified crops and the poisonous substances used to harvest them are disrupting the soil. Countless chemicals are used on GM crops. When applying weed and fungicide killers to crops, this creates super weeds and superbugs (plants and bugs resistant to these chemicals). The bugs and weeds naturally and unnaturally become resistant to the chemicals and this can wreak havoc.

This resistance creates a host of new types of concerns for crop harvesting. It could assist bacteria and insects in their ability to potentially morph, adapt, and resist death. As humans, we already have enough of a load trying to protect and sanitize the human body. We don't need more superbugs or super-resistant bacteria to come into the picture.

Unhealthy fabric finishing treatments

Flame-retardant fabric: PBDE diphenyl ether, a neurotoxin and endocrine disruptor, is found in chemical-treated, flame-retardant fabric finishes. PBDEs have also been found in breast milk, house dust, and laundry lint traps. Flame-retardant textile finishes in apparel are not very useful. The odds of catching on fire are rare. Even so, these flame-retardant fabrics are not exactly fireproof and could never protect the wearer against a natural fire in a similar way to a firefighter's outfit. The chemicals in fire-retardant fabrics of daily wear work against the body. Catching on fire shouldn't be a major concern, it just gives us a reason to douse fabrics with more toxic poisons.

Attapulgite clay can be used as a natural, alternative, healthy flame-retardant fabric treatment and finish. Studies have shown "outstanding fire-retardant properties" in non-toxic attapulgite clay. It's a useful and important alternative to chemically-treated, flame-retardant fabrics.

Formaldehyde: Formaldehyde fumes can leak out when wearing and washing garments made with an anti-wrinkle, formaldehyde fabric treatment. The International Agency for Research on Cancer declares formaldehyde to be a carcinogen. Side-effects caused by its use include nausea, breathing difficulties, and seizures, among others. We could add natural ingredients to detergents, and develop more plant-based fabric softeners and new finishing treatments to help keep fabrics from wrinkling.

Silver-treated fabrics: Silver-treated fabrics are promoted as an antifungal treatment, yet the coatings and amount of silver make this detrimental to health. Because it's antibacterial, the microbial silver finish of germ-repelling clothing is counterproductive, as it can disrupt the healthy flora that is part of the skin's acid mantle.

The silver can leach onto the body's cells. Nano-silver is shed from fabric when skin sweats or when fabric is rubbed against the skin. The size of this finish is nano-molecular, small enough to be absorbed through the surface layer of the skin or inhaled through the mouth.

Too much silver will cause metal poisoning, and in this case, potentially argyria, where the skin turns blue. A man used a colloidal silver formula internally and topically on his skin for many years. His face and body eventually turned a permanent shade of blue.

Along with the above effects, when silver-based fabrics are laundered, the silver-finishes and/or silver threads break down in the laundry, moving into waterways, damaging and threatening sea life. The silver nanoparticles are found in waste and water systems, and are then absorbed into the skin through drinking water.

Synthetic and animal textile dyes

Vijayakumar Varathan used to mix chemicals in a conventional textile factory for decades. He developed a skin disease which made layers of his skin peel off. He decided to begin working with plant-based dyes instead. Unfortunately, his skin to this day is permanently damaged from synthetic dyes.

Synthetic dyes are almost completely made of petrochemicals. Roughly 60–70% of all chemical dyes are azo-based dyes. Azo dyes are carcinogenic and mutagenic. The waste streams of dye baths are toxic, making waterways unsuitable to drink from, or bathe in. We can make dyes with non-toxic chemicals. Not all chemicals have to be made toxic.

Textile dyes made of bacteria

Bacteria-dyed textiles to replace synthetic dyes could lead to skin infections, among other issues. Various bacteria types may not be hygienic to wear. Studies have shown that certain bacteria pigments can cause infection. A few bacteria types used and tested to produce colored dye are *P. aeruginosa* and *E. coli*. *E. coli* produces a blue dye known as indigoidine. Scientists created a biosynthetic gene manipulation to produce large amounts of dye color from bacteria for textile use. We already have both healthy and sometimes non-healthy flora flourishing on the surface of our skin. Additional foreign bacteria exposed to skin doesn't prove to be a harmonious addition and can cause interference to the body and the skin's acid mantle.

Animal dyes

Tyrian purple comes from the ink of a sea snail. When attacked or threatened, snails spray a purple ink. The mollusk is crushed to obtain the ink for dyeing. This life-form could easily be left in its natural habitat. Another example is the use of bugs. Cochineal, a semi-popular natural dye, is made from squashed insects. There are ethical ways of collecting cochineal bugs when they are dead, to extract the color. Even so, bugs in general are not the most hygienic dye substance to use.

Synthetic fabrics are bacteria producing

The highest bacterial growth-forming fabrics are polyester, nylon, acrylic, and wool. A synthetic fabric's bacterial growth is formed when the bacteria germinates in heat. Synthetic fabric doesn't readily absorb or wick sweat, making it easy for bacteria to settle onto the skin's surface. Even when a synthetic fabric has technical wick-performing properties, they still keep sweat locked in and on the surface of the skin.

It doesn't matter what fabrics we have on; we are going to sweat in it eventually. But plant-based fabrics still allow the skin to breathe while the skin sweats. Natural, plant-based fabrics are gently antimicrobial and antibacterial, leaving the fabric and skin with less ability to create excess bacterial growth. Skin has millions of bacteria. The microbiota of skin repels the disease-producing microbes. However, healthy bacteria can also multiply to an unhealthy degree and wreak havoc on skin and the immune system.

People are much more prone to infection when bacterial growth occurs. Most people are immune-deficient based on nutrient deficiency, stress, and environmental pollution, among numerous other causes. If a person can develop a cold or flu, they are immune-deficient. Colds and flus are infections. Unbalanced pH fabrics can discourage and aggravate the acid mantle, driving the skin to produce more bacteria, and this will affect our immune system.

The skin's acid mantle can become a breeding ground for external foreign matter. If fabrics and human skin are not clean enough, they can spread unwanted germs, bacteria and support a virus. Common bacteria types naturally present in skin do not harm the body in small bacterial count numbers. What is often overlooked, however, are the types of bacteria that develop issues when overproduced.

Pathogen/toxicity of micrococci

Studies have shown that synthetic fabrics carry the most abundant growth of micrococci. Micrococci are related to coryne bacteria, members of the actinobacteria phylum. Micrococci bacteria on polyester were highest in abundance, and none were found in cotton. Micrococci emit malodor, producing a toxic smell. Micrococci are not found in large quantities on human skin, making it evident that the synthetic fabric is producing the bacterial overgrowth. Immune-deficient people pick up infection from micrococci more easily. Systemic conditions caused by micrococci include pulmonary hemorrhage, septic shock, pneumonia, urinary infection, immune deficiency, and more.

Lyocell, the hypoallergenic, regenerated wood-based fabric, retains a very low, bacterial growth count. A study concluded that bacterial growth rate increases up to 2,000 times in synthetic fabric. The humidity control property restricts lyocell from growing bacteria. It is an antibacterial, odor-preventing fabric. Lyocell preventatively reduces bacterial overgrowth partly based on its fibril-like composition and its material. It locks moisture inside the material and releases it onto the fabric's outer surface to evaporate.

Bacterial growth can be managed through optimal laundering care, yet it can still be an issue even with proper laundering. Infection and bacteria can spread fairly fast. Additionally, coats, jackets, hats, shoes, scarves, bags, and uniforms are not regularly laundered. Activewear, too, can harbor toxic bacteria. The bacteria can then leach and grow on the skin. Bacteria may become embedded and it does not always simply wash off with water.

Synthetic fabrics promote infection

In the medical field, doctors prescribe natural cotton underwear over synthetic underwear if one carries an infection of any sort, like a female's vaginal yeast infection, or a male's groin infection. Synthetic fabrics trap in heat and sweat. When they create excess moisture, the infection breeds and persists. Plant-based fabrics have the potential to help treat not only external, but internal infection and more widespread skin infections, even when they are bred internally beneath the skin tissue.

Petroleum-based plastic menstrual pads are a very obvious example of plastic irritating the skin. A lot of menstrual pads, the ones produced for female menstruation, are full of plastic. One single pad can contain up to four disposable shopping plastic bags worth of plastic. Plastic pads have been found to trap in heat and dampness, and reduce air flow in the groin area, leading to chronic yeast infections, vaginal irritations, and allergies.

Overall, the use of gentle, antibacterial fabrics and fabric treatments prevents bacteria from breeding on fabrics and the skin. Fabric finishes must work with the skin's acid mantle and pH in order to resist an immune disorder and/or skin issue. The focus should be on gentle, cleansing fabric treatments like aloe, castor oil, and plant dyes with naturally occurring antibacterial properties that are efficient in promoting healthy skin.

Animal-based fabrics and materials: their disadvantages

This section discusses the negative qualities of animal-based materials. Animal-based apparel is controversial. Not all animal-derived fashion materials are created equal. Some are genuinely acceptable and healthy, yet in other cases, we might be better off without them. Generally speaking, they are better than synthetic fabrics because they are natural and not synthetically made. Yet, synthetic fabrics are better than animal-based fibers because there's no ethical way they can clothe the masses entirely. In minor quantities they are needed at this time, until there is widespread demand for all-weather plant-based fabrics.

Addressing the issues concerning animal-based fashion is not supposed to raise any form of political argument about them. Some people would say it is not good to wear; however, Native Americans wore animal-based fashion in a sacred way, extensively. It was a part of the Native Americans' survival, and that's respectable. They honored and respected animal life. Based on their extreme wisdom, their use of plant-medicine, and the values of their culture, their traditions are effectively modern for this day and age.

There may always be animal-based fashion. Native Americans made it ethical, yet it needs to be kept and maintained as a niche market. For the sake of survival, it is unrealistic to boycott animal-based fashion entirely at this point in time. The problem is that animal-derived clothing has been exploited simply through excessive use. It is not the most fitting for the future of fashion if used in excess.

Animal-based fabrics are used predominantly for cold-climate weather. They offer protective, thermal properties. Regardless, it is not the most essential or beneficial apparel product of choice. Synthetic, petroleum-based fabric should be the first textile to go before animal fibers, but animal fibers are not a replacement.

Holistic methods of animal production are available. There are several small, local, and culturally acceptable organizations, using traditional and sustainable methods of producing animal-based textiles, with a balanced production cycle. These humane organizations and artisanal production practices are non-exploitative.

It is impractical and non-sustainable to produce animal fiber products on a mass surplus scale. Minimal use of animal products in the fashion industry creates more ethical choices and boundaries for humane animal treatment. Exploitation in animal farming has increased to an unnatural extent. More and more, textile markets are using soon-to-be slaughtered animals from the food industry. About 90% of those farms are not raising organic-fed or free-range animals.

A significant portion of the food industry is inhumane in its approach to animal farming, with mistreatment of animals throughout the rearing process and right up to their death. It's highly unusual for mass animal-rearing farms to allow natural death. The horrors of roadkill are much more prolifically felt by people than the horrors of animal slaughter and butcher-house death.

There is animal abuse in the fur, leather, and feather industry. More and more brands are turning away from these types of materials. Animal skin is no longer appearing luxurious. Animals are used in a negative way when plucked and skinned alive. Their tails, tusks, and ears are cut off. They are caged until they are of no use to humanity. When there is no more room for them to breathe, they are killed.

Additionally, wearing animal products may not be hygienic. Animals are subjected to bugs, insects, larvae, bacteria, microbes, and fungus that cannot simply be washed away. It's embedded in the material. Most fabric treatments and cleaning solvents cannot be used to thoroughly sanitize animal-based fabrics, as they are too harsh, and would destroy the material itself.

The negative effects of wearing wool

A particular issue with wool is the dryness and high static that occurs when it's worn. Wool is ranked highest for static because it's a conductive material. This moisture loss is caused by the wool fibers' hollow structure. The fact that it is a conductive fiber makes it create uncomfortable static and skin dryness. It induces static which accumulates debris, making the wool attract and accumulate lint on fabric very easily.

Wool tends to have a different reaction to collecting moisture because it does not have an absorbent, hollow structure like plant fibers do. Moisture on the skin gets trapped in the fiber, on the front, back and surface of the fabric, resulting in clammy skin. When sweat is collected on wool, the fibers and skin feel more wet, when compared to plant fibers that absorb the sweat more, keeping the body more dry.

Many wool textiles are rough, causing skin abrasion, stressing the skin. Other wool textiles are soft, yet still give off an itchy, prickly feeling. Superfine merino wool has the lowest micron count of any wool textile and does not give rise to a prickly sensation. Apart from merino wool and cashmere, most wool fabrics touch the skin's surface and trigger nerves and nerve endings. The nociceptors in the skin, which are pain stimuli reactors, are triggered. This is tactile interference. There are ways to produce a comfortable wool product. Wearing a wool product as an outer layer is a way to stay warm, and for certain cases like extreme weather. Overall, though, wool is not the most suitable fabric due to its irritant factors. If a person is tactile tolerant to it, it can be an option.

Wool cannot be bleached because bleach has a high pH. Bleach is extremely alkaline and dissolves the animal hair, turning it into a yellowish, felted material. Additionally, wool and other animal fibers felt in hot water, making the garment useless due to shrinkage. Also, the newly felted fabric thus irritates skin. Wool is not as easy to clean because you can't dry it in the dryer or use hot water. Hot water or garment drying is used in conjunction with detergents to destroy bacteria, dust, and other foreign particles nested into the fabric.

Animal-based fabrics do not have antibacterial properties like plant-based fabrics do. Wool, for instance, is stripped of its natural emollient, lanolin, which makes wool more antibacterial. Wool products are high-growth, bacterial carriers. A study revealed that MRSA (methicillin-resistant staphylococcus aureus) survived on wool longer than any other fabric. Wool may be odor-reducing, but it does not eliminate the bacteria itself. Takashima's study states that wool, polyester, and acrylic can be carriers of the bacteria S. aureus. S. aureus is one of the most disease-causing bacteria, causing bloodstream infections, pneumonia, and bone and joint infections.

Studies reveal that animal products are hypoallergenic, but many people have allergic-type reactions to wool. Wool may trap dust and foreign particles. It also can't keep foreign particles from irritating and agitating skin. Wool acts as a filter; therefore soil, debris, bacteria, and air-pollutants are trapped, as they nest and burrow, within wool. This is similar to a kitchen dish sponge. It may clean dishes with hot water and frothy soap, but the sponge itself locks in the dirty bacteria and microbes.

Fabric pests are much more drawn to wool, silk and leather. Most wool and silk attract moths, silverfish, beetles, and mold that can live in a garment and ultimately destroy it. Bug infestations, particularly in wool and silk, can occur at any time, and not only when they are left in the closet over time. Most plant-based fabrics do not have this issue, but some bugs will eat plant-based fibers.

Leather

Leather lasts and doesn't damage easily, so it's sustainable in this way. It was ethically produced in Native American cultures. Leather is kept in its place in luxury industry circles due to its everlasting life-cycle. Plant-based materials do not contain genetic material like human DNA, that's closely linked with animal DNA. So, they are cleaner fabrics and naturally hygienic, compared with a material derived from an animal's own personal DNA, and contain dead cells and foreign matter. Additionally, there's an epidemic of toxic tannins used in the tanning of leathers, and this is causing negative symptoms among the leather industry workers and leather wearers.

Another consideration is the energy of leather. Everything is made up of energy, and death energy may be a part of leather. Dead skin can potentially harbor feelings of fear, anger, and sadness. The scientist and author, Masuro Emoto, was able to prove this. He created a crystallization test for the effect of human consciousness on the structure of water molecules. One of Emoto's water crystal experiments: a jar of water was embraced with feelings of love before it was frozen. When it was taken out of the freezer, the crystallized water formation looked beautiful, with intricate sacred geometric patterns. The water molecules displayed a deformed, fragmented imprint after a jar of water was being subjected to emotions of fear, hate, and anger. Similarly, due to an animal's life and death experience, leather could naturally harbor animals' negative energy and negative emotions.

Ethics of fur

It is one thing when Native Americans in the dead of winter found it necessary for their survival to hunt and gather food and animal-based materials to stay warm. Animal skin and fur were beneficial to them. They were used in their homes, clothing and shelter. However, in this day and age, mass hunting, killing, and breeding of furs is considered animal exploitation. Apparently, we have not continued the Native Americans' sacred approach towards their animal-based clothing. Earth is advancing as a culture where other forms of technology are available and killing animals is not necessary to stay warm.

Silk

Silk is not especially hygienic if you consider what it is actually made up of. It's made of a protein fiber, fibroin, that is secreted from silkworms. Silkworms are the offspring of moths. While the bugs flip around constantly, they secrete a chemical out of their mouths. The chemical secretion is used to build their cocoon. The silk fibroin is spun and made into silk fabric. So wearing silk is like wearing bugs: their juices. Also, imagine the type of energy that's embedded in this fabric, as the bug is constantly jerking its body in the cocoon in order for it to develop. Bugs don't belong on the exterior of the skin. Additionally, there is negative tactile, and negative sensorial activity coming off of silk.

Animal farming

About 70 billion farm animals are raised for food in the world each year. To make groundbreaking elevations of consciousness on this planet, we need to decrease animal farming for fashion and apparel and increase the rise of plant-based fashion.

Many would declare there is huge gain for the fashion industry to use animal products. Not only do we use animals for their meat, but also for our clothes. However, animal breeding can be taken to an extreme. Ultimately, the more animals used, the less ethical the process, and more exploitation arises. Factoring in the breeding of genetically altered animals, mass farming of animals, and unethically altering their DNA for purposes that are not all clear, we can see there are nonbeneficial aspects of animal-based clothing.

The biotech of genetically engineered animals

Lab-grown leathers are made from the DNA taken from animal skin. The leathers are made into fabrics without using the animal itself; only a small sample of their DNA is needed to replicate them. Silk without worms, leather without cows, fur without rabbits. One lab leather method manipulates the animal hide cell through a bioreactor. It uses 3D bioprinting cell formation.

Another issue arises here, with breeding hybrid animals by altering their DNA. For example, scientists have created transgenic spider-goats that make a silk-like fabric, also named BioSteel™, from their milk. A scientist put a spider's dragline gene into a goat in order for it to produce goat/spider silk threads to be made into fabric. Creating goat/spider hybrids is not humane, and can further complicate things.

Mutating animals could open up a can of worms, and it's unhealthy. It could potentially cause animal mutations that affect the Earth. Several researchers and textile manufacturers are more and more interested in replicating spider silk. The production of spider silk is like a robotic science. It's a part of a negative, transhumanist regime, but with animals. This could, unfortunately, get more popular, and unnatural chaos will result.

Human leather made from human skin is in development and has been produced. Bear in mind, there is no current law or regulation for protecting one's own DNA for commercialization. There are immoral ramifications of wearing lab-generated human skin leather taken from dead corpses, or living persons. There are real risks involved, posing a threat to physical and psychological health. To use animal leather as a proposition to ultimately blur the lines between animal leather and human leather is not healthy. Additionally, it seems unethical, unacceptable, and unhygienic.

Chapter 6

Unhealthy Fashion Technologies

Greenwashing demystified

Greenwash myth 1: Synthetic fabric is sustainable

It's a misconstrued idea that synthetic fabric is sustainable. A synthetic fabric may be considered sustainable when its life cycle is prolonged, but it still cannot be considered sustainable as they don't adhere to a circular model. In any context, it cannot be labeled a sustainable option, because eventually it ends up in the landfill, taking up to 200 years before it breaks down and decomposes. Even if it's regenerated multiple times it has an end point, and you can't compost it, because it's a non-biodegradable material.

Naturally, when you think of the word "sustainable," you think "healthy." Several synthetic fabrics and products are labeled sustainable, making people perceive them as healthy. Some companies call themselves sustainable yet offer a ton of synthetic garments. It's deceptive to conceal synthetic fabrics and their toxic properties. A little synthetic fabric is OK, people need to survive. But these manufacturers and brands are using misleading advertising and supporting a material that's not beneficial for humans or the environment. When a company is not fully aware of the negative health effects of these fabrics, it's all too easy for that company to suggestively call its products "sustainable."

There has recently been a rise of synthetic fibers blended with plant-based fibers, and these fabric blends are produced for greater profit. It is still better to wear blended fabrics made with both plant and synthetic fibers than wear a 100% synthetic garment; however, there needs to be a rise of 100%

plant-based fabric fashions. These plant/synthetic fiber blends are deceiving the consumer and making it difficult to detect if a fabric is natural or synthetic, because often its texture feels like cotton. Fabric technology can make synthetic fabric look and feel like ergonomic natural fibers, but it's a scam.

Masking the synthetic material, and mocking it as a plant-based material in order to make it reach consumer demand, proves what the customer wants: a plant-based garment. They are better than 100% synthetic fabrics, but realistically they cannot perform sustainably or be a complete healing modality. Additionally, only partial biodegradation of these fabrics occurs, and you can't compost them.

If synthetic textile designers and synthetic textile manufacturers are imitating the qualities of cotton and linen, this reveals that they acknowledge plant-based fabric as superior to synthetic fabric. People are usually genuinely interested in creating a healthy product, but the high demand for synthetic fabrics creates a lack of plant-based fabric demand. Businesses and consumers are being driven to make decisions based on currently technology and what's being currently produced.

Greenwash myth 2: Recycled polyester made from plastic bottles is sustainable

Among the current eco fashion trends is the production of recycled plastic bottles being turned into fabrics. This recycled plastic fabric is considered sustainable as it keeps the bottles from piling up in landfills. If plastic bottles don't belong in landfills, they certainly don't belong on the body.

To give a toxic substance like plastic bottles more lifespan, only to continue its toxic disruption through apparel, this is not sustainable fashion. It's supporting the continued production of plastic. Recycled plastic bottle fabric will end up in the landfill taking up to 450 years to decompose. If it's not sustainable for the Earth, it won't be for the body, and vice versa. There's no use to defend it unless it's biodegradable, biobased plastic. An alternative to plastic is hemp plastic, or other bioplastics.

Ocean plastic trash and recycled plastic bottles used to make apparel will cause more microplastic pollution and a poisoned food supply chain. Plastic builds up in the digestive tract of sea creatures. If plastic is a threat to sea life, it could also be a cause for concern to wear plastic fabric. Human existence as part of the ecological system needs to be brought more into the picture.

Recycled plastic bottle fabric is not healthy. For one, not all plastic is BPA-free. BPA disrupts the endocrine and hormone system. Even through a BPA extraction process, the bisphenol is not removed and it's as equally toxic as BPA. Skin doesn't work like the liver; it doesn't filter toxins. When the body is heated or sweating, the chemicals from the fabrics and dyes can leach into the skin. They go through the skin into the bloodstream and spread throughout the body systems. As conscious consumers, we must be aware of how synthetic fabric technology may be a distraction from what the material is actually made from: a petroleum by-product.

Greenwash myth 3: Rubber is healthy to wear

Petroleum-based rubber, also named latex, is a greenwashed material and not healthy for topical use. It's used in apparel, fabric, jewelry, bags, shoes, and surf apparel. Several companies are using recycled car tires for accessories and shoes. A smell of toxic fumes permeates from the rubber. Rubber in general is not the best thing to wear for topical use as it's not breathable.

In general, rubber is filled with toxic chemicals, carcinogens and heavy metals that release toxic fumes and outgas residue. When burned, it releases harmful chemicals like benzene, polycyclic aromatic hydrocarbons (PAHS), and styrene.

Alternative sources of plant-based rubbers can come from plants such as trees and dandelions.

Greenwash myth 4: Nanotextiles are healthy

Nanotextiles are a relatively new trend in the textile industry. There are fabrics that have nanoparticles, nanofibers, nanofilaments, and/or nanowires built into the yarn/fibers, or sprayed on as a coated fabric finishing treatment. Nanoparticles are built in the yarn/fiber of a textile. Nanocapsule fabric treatments are built into the finishing, coating, and additive treatments of a fabric.

The main issue of nanotechnology is the lack of safeguards, evaluation, and testing done to prove that these products are safe. None of the nano-based coatings and finishes need to be labeled on any tag or certified. It's pretty evident that not all nanoparticles are natural or plant-derived, some are synthetic and artificially made.

Many of the materials used are toxic and synthetic, so, the materials of the nanocapsule itself need to be assessed, along with the ingredients within the capsule. These microcapsules need to be non-toxic and plant-derived. Also, they should be filled with gentle, non-potent, plant-derived ingredients.

Nanotextiles include ingredients with potential risks such as oxide/hydroxide, phosphate, metal sulfide, carbonaceous NP, metal oxide, and more. In some cases, nanomaterials have the ability to grow, morph, and be artificially alive, a function that might simply be invasive. Because of their size, they could penetrate into the skin and orifices.

Silver nanoparticles, and titanium dioxide nanoparticles used in "sunscreen fabrics" pose health risks. These metals are not regulated. One nanotextile fabric treatment is a carbon nanotube coating, used for its thermoregulation property. A study from the University of Edinburgh found that carbon nanotubes one billionth of an atom wide reacted in the lungs of mice. This was likened to asbestos, which causes a lethal lung cancer.

There are several negative ailments associated with nanoparticle exposure. Animal studies have shown that through lung inhalation, nanoparticles are harmful, and can result in pulmonary effects such as inflammation, fibrosis, and carcinogenicity. Some nanomaterials have proved to be toxic to human tissue and body cells, and they increase oxidative stress.

Only a few scientific developments of nanoscience have been approved by the FDA. If people are already finding risks of nanoparticles ingested by fish and nature, it is evident that they could affect the health of humans. Additionally, the health effects of nanoparticles interacting with the environment are not entirely clear either, but this new technology can easily pose a threat to natural habitats. Studies have shown that nanoparticles can be used as transporters and carriers of pathogens and other toxic substances.

Unhealthy apparel and accessories that suppress and restrict the body

Worldwide, since ancient times, fashion industry regimes have possessed people to mutilate their own body to some degree. When sacrificial attire takes hold over someone, ergonomic fashion is not an option. Body modification in fashion is a concern, and a pressure put on society.

Traditional styles of dress that modify the body can still be worn for costume and occasion wear. Temporary use won't necessarily threaten anyone's life; however, there are still many physically and mentally punishing fashion products being produced that shouldn't be worn at all.

An example of a fashion/beauty body modification is foot binding, which dates back to the tenth century in China. In Asia, tight foot binding disfigured and crushed the female foot until it became "petite." The toes were wrapped tightly around the sole of the foot. One woman from China was forced to bind her foot over and over until all her toes, and the tendons and arch in her foot, were broken. This woman currently has no feeling in her feet.

The girl's parents forced her to bind her feet, and threatened her, telling her she would never marry if she didn't have small feet. Yet, foot binding was really practiced to keep young girls and women still, so that they would be kept to work on crafts like mats, yarn, fiber, cloth, and shoe-making. Foot binding is now illegal, but you would be surprised at the amount of body-modifications around the world that are still being used today for the sake of "beauty."

In Africa, a neck brace binds the neck to manipulate its desired length to the point where the neck piece cannot be taken off; complications and fatality may occur as the neck can no longer hold the head up. Corsets, originating in Europe, are another form of body mutilation as they can morph, crack, and fracture ribs. The organs are bruised, become distorted, and shift.

Belts are a modern form of the girdle. They are detrimental to health if not worn properly. Belts cause shallow breathing because they are mostly made of leather or plastic materials without any give. You can't really wear a belt without it squeezing something. Increased or normal lung capacity requires belly breathing. When one's breath is held or there is breath obstruction, it can become irregular, challenging the body. Anything too tight-fitting around the stomach can result in acid reflux, digestive issues, organ suppression, and nerve irritation.

If people want to wear a belt, stretch-knit belts will help the belly breathe, producing ease and flow. Elastic is good, but it all depends on its tension. Belts are a major accessory item that can elevate a look, but ergonomic belts should be chosen.

High heels should ideally be worn only as occasion wear. Heels cause vulnerability by impairing a person's physical motion, making them accident prone. They can hurt the foot, causing slight to severe injury. Ergonomic high heel shoes should have grip and shock resistance to improve their performance.

Compression garments/contour-shaping garments

Some compression garments are beneficial. They support weakened, stretched-out organs and help stimulate blood circulation. However, this really depends on its fabric technology, design, and how and where it is placed on the body. Some contour-shaping garments lift areas of the body that should not be lifted or squeezed. They are controlling the body, making it appear more lifted and firm. The body generally needs to flow, yet some measures of constriction can be effective. Fitted clothing that hugs the body can support the flow and movement of the body, just as much as the ease of less-fitted clothes that support flow and movement.

Suppression can occur from cage-like, underwire bras constricting breath. Metal should not be a material used to support the breast area. This is a form of body manipulation. Underwire bras are being linked with a host of cancer-afflicted conditions. They also pose a risk to child-bearing women. Underwire materials are too hard. The hard materials used put an unnecessary, increased pressure that conflicts with this sensitive area. Bras should be made of natural materials and stretch-based fabrics to appropriately protect and support this sensitive area. There are plenty of ergonomic designs and technical developments that can support the breast area, while also supporting lung function.

Extra-fitted fashion designs made from woven, non-stretch fabrics

Tight-fitting clothing is another health issue. Woven apparel, in general, is not stretchy. They can be movement-restricting based on a garment's construction, fit, and cut, and it's something to watch out for. All woven materials can be adjusted to support the body. Sheath dresses made without stretch constrict the body, causing fainting and oxygen deprivation. A fitted dress may need to be made with stretch-knit fabric to ease tightness.

Business suiting, for example, is particularly restricting. They keep a person from moving around. Blazers and suit jackets can be tight and ill-fitting, not meant for performance and movement. Skirts with non-stretch waistbands can act like restricting belts. When polyester blouses have tightly-buttoned cuffs, and lined skirts and jackets are made with woven fabric and have less give, the wearer will experience exasperation. The body systems can eventually shut down, making us become immobile, exhausted.

The issues of certain digital fashion tech

This is the digital age, and technology is fast. The fashion industry attempts to keep up to speed with digital technology itself. However, fashion cannot contend with the internet in terms of its speed. Technology serves the purpose of human advancement, but we are not meant to replicate its speed. Part of the fashion industry is being set up to become a manmade, robotic technology, not to bring about Earth's natural rhythms. There are setbacks when people believe that we should adapt or imitate a machinist system. Too much digital-influenced fashion is caused by humanity's disconnect from Earth and the repercussions are: living a synthetic lifestyle. Andy Goldsworthy stated: "We often forget that we are nature. Nature is not something separate from us. So, when we have lost our connection to nature, we have lost our connection to ourselves."

In today's modern world, society is amidst creating a balancing act between a natural and urban lifestyle. Using digital fashion to administer healthy solutions without it being disruptive to communities and individuals is a promising development. Tech programs and social media can be misused. Digital advertisements can become manipulative. The industry's current digital modes of operation must be taken into account for the health of future generations. Providing safe outlets and holistic digital contributions will inspire people to have balance between nature and tech, in their lifestyle.

Wearable tech

There are already enough tech accessories like cellphones and computers emitting radiation that people are subjected to. Digital fashion accessories are an unnecessary addition, unless it's a health monitor or used temporarily. However, fashion accessories such as computer watches placed directly on the skin can interfere with the body's natural electronic circuit.

Computer watches are connected to satellites emitting levels of carcinogenic radiation. The human aura is a protective barrier that works to ward off radiation. Cellphones and laptops aren't strapped to the body, so there is a difference when we place digital products directly on the body and human aura.

Research has been conducted to study the real hazards of these devices. The electronic devices were reported to be inducing cancer, tumors, and blood problems. Scientists are calling some EMFs a "slow poison." A WHO panel, with over 31 scientists in 14 countries, concluded that cellphones are possibly carcinogenic, and as toxic as chemicals and pesticides.

New and more wearable tech products will be available as the tech industry continues to rise. Digital garments, internet-connected glasses, and other devices are a few other examples of new, relevant tech products that are directly exposed to the skin and should not be used.

The RFID chip technology used in apparel

The RFID (radio frequency identification) chip or tag is a technology system and a growing trend in fashion retail management. It's a surveillance system used to track merchandise, control inventory, reduce counterfeit, and limit theft.

Corporate retailers, department stores, and high-profile brands typically use RFID technology. The pros are that censored chips prevent theft, and companies can track their inventory without even opening shipped boxes. Inventory and sold-out products are quickly detected, making it easy to trace their product.

RFID chips are typically placed on the side-seams of apparel. They need to be cut off at the time of purchase. Not all chips will get recognized, however, as some are embedded into the fabric. Some are small enough to be lodged within yarn, while some are implanted in the sole of a shoe. There's no easy, distinguishable way to prove clothing is chipped when they're hidden. Most chips are washable and waterproof. Additionally, on the production end, assembling carcinogenic chips is hazardous to humans. Another consideration is its end use. Chips don't biodegrade, which affects the ecosystem.

There are unethical aspects of RFID chip installation in apparel. It can be used to surveil people. People may need to approach it as a legal matter, because it's a privacy threat. As it is wired to satellite and radio wave technology, the RFID chip can involuntarily be operated in additional systems that use chip software, that are separate from the chip's original source.

So, the company itself operating the RFID chip system may not be interested in surveilling a person, but because of its technology, it is a worldwide, satellite-operated venture, giving the RFID chip the ability to connect to other systems/programs as an open circuit for secretive, operative communication. This suggests the chip software can be used for control, similar to the way totalitarian governments have acted towards entire populations.

The RFID chip itself has been called the "mark of the beast." There's been mention of people being chipped in order for the government to establish more control over its people. If our clothes have a permanently embedded RFID chip in them, and we wear these clothes all the time, it may just be another form of control.

The medical industry is chipping patients in order to recover their medical history faster. Also, companies around the world chip their employees, and some of these implants are used to access the company's building. Chips are also being injected in train ride customers, to pay for their train rides more easily.

A problem with this chip device system is it's attached to the product, thus interfering with the body. It's a health hazard as it's connected to a radiation-emitting antenna. RFID chips, when worn topically, emit an unnatural frequency current to the body.

Studies show, RFID chip implants pose health risks to humans and animals. RFID chips on clothing are like chip implants embedded under skin, and could potentially be, or are, utilized in that way. A chip placed in fabric or on clothing may not be injected under the skin, but because it is a carrier near and direct to the skin's surface it can have similar, negative side effects like that of an injected chip.

Many reports of RFID chipped pets and animals describe symptoms of limb weakness, cancer, and other issues. Removing the chip may not be achievable if a chip migrates in the body. Constant exposure to radiation happens when the RFID chip is worn internally or externally. Many animal tests have shown they cause tumors and cysts that surround the chip itself. A lab study at Dow Chemical Company in the 1990s revealed that RFID chips induced tumors in mice and rats. The tumors were encapsulating the glass-encased transponder chip.

In some countries—in parts of Europe, for example—many

of their retail stores are asked to relay to the customer that there is a chip tag sewn within the garment, and that it needs to be clipped off. Most places do not need to disclose this information, however, because there are very few regulations involved.

Skin tissue can evidently react to chips. It's like microwave radiation. It can burn and aggravate the skin if not removed. For example, a burning, stinging sensation on the skin occurs when a person holds a cellphone for too long. The chip gives off the same burning sensation. No company should use the RFID chip system if it will threaten the wearer. This technology will evidently backfire.

Artificial intelligence in fashion

One fashion tech development is using artificial intelligence to compute the statistics of current trends via algorithm. This data is used to create clothing hybrids. The algorithms of a garment, and its color, silhouette, shape, cut, size, that are most purchased and on-trend can be manipulated and morphed and used in other designs for the likelihood of increased sales. This is like artificial engineering versus going the natural route of recreating and slightly altering a design's original form via natural adaptation. The natural route is more authentic.

Artificial intelligence tech creates collective data pools to drive technology further. The collected data can resurface trends and compute what's new based on pools of information. Programs collect data from fashion shows of hundreds of designers and pick up on trends, artificially migrating them for more selling power and more conversion within a given population.

Artificial intelligence technologies can ultimately try to manipulate the natural, intuitive-based fashion forecasting. Depending on the direction this will take fashion, a balance of intuition and the creative process is necessary to foster authentic growth within trend markets.

Fashion forecasting is an intuitive, creative process. Both the industry and consumers participate. When the fashion industry is naturally in rhythm with the pace of life, Earth evolves.

Chapter 7

Unhealthy Fashion for Mind, Body, and Spirit

.

Exploitation in fashion

Body exploitation in fashion; embracing body image in fashion

Fashion is exploited worldwide. Body exploitation in fashion is negative connotation, sexual suggestion, and violence that is detrimentally expressed through fashion in a variety of ways. Clothing can be used to manipulate and intentionally control, inducing fear. Choosing to accept the body through healthy ways of dressing will help keep people from using clothing as a weapon.

Clothing is a tool to protect the body, not for entertaining negative behaviors. Using fashion for protection disrupts fashion used as a control mechanism. A good example of cultures embracing body image and removing body exploitation is the launch of the legging trend, which was driven by the athleisure trend. Leggings are a positive tool for empowerment and social equality. They stand for purpose. The legging trend proves to be a healthy way to accept the human body, as they empower women to embrace their body shape. Wherever body discrimination is welcomed, leggings can be worn, as they take a stand for body acceptance.

Leggings are a model product for daily attire, and can be worn both as a trend and as a classic. Leggings are fitted, come in different fabric weights and can be worn with every and any top imaginable. They are aerodynamic, move with the body, and are a style staple They are comfortable, ergonomic, and easy to wear, which is partly why they are so trendy.

Women of all ages are wearing leggings, making them an age-defying product. The legging trend diffuses the judgement of a person by their age. It is a style that turns against age discrimination that is rooted from a false fashion perception. Age is all about attitude and style. Leggings infiltrate every age and every body shape. This creates less segregation and less deception. There is a universal need for age acceptance. Fashion becomes modern when it is utilized as a method that creates age acceptance, yet all the while creating a more youthful culture.

The legging trend, because it embraces all ages and body types, is a necessary remedy against superficial attire with sexual connotations that exploit the body.

Body parts can be exposed, it's not always an act of seduction. There are tribal populations dressed half-naked or completely naked, adorned only with jewelry. This is culturally acceptable, not offensive, because it's done with the wearer's authentic intention, and because of their culture's apparel use customs. Additionally, swimwear and activewear help neutralize the perception of clothing that is sometimes expressed negatively or expressed in a sexually perverse way. Healthy fashion is not provocative fashion; neither does it revolt against the genuineness of the human body.

Sexual exploitation; creating healthy boundaries through clothing

Throughout the generations, and in many parts of the world, people have been desensitized by fashion and the exploitative use of apparel used as a weapon. Misguided use of clothing can result in women and men being observed as objects. Self-objectification is a person who treats themselves as an object, and they are to be perceived and judged by their appearance. Superficial, artificial clothing tends to exhibit the body as an object. Clothing holistically encompassing the body to express the spirit and soul within is non-objectified fashion.

Apart from the legging trend being modern and body-accepting, they can appear derogatory or used to attract male attention. This is not about the leggings anymore; it's about the women in their body portraying leggings as sexual. People's energy and body language can create sexual connotations that are inappropriate and disrespectful. People's energy body and language can relay a type of false awareness of sexual objectification in misguided fashion.

Sexually explicit, derogatory clothing is clothing misused for control and power. It is not really the clothing's fault. Neither is it the fault of the person's interpretation of the wearer's misguided dress; people do not want to slander another person's way of dress. However, it's a natural, instinctive reaction to be provoked by this type of dress. Whether a person is conscious of wearing misguided clothing or not, it is the wearer's fault if their intention is not pure and they misuse fashion.

Another woman could be wearing the same sexually exploitative outfit and manage to look respectful, not expressing lust or looking like she's revealing her body in a sexual way. It is a matter of a person's attitude, how clothing is being worn, and how they represent themselves by their presence, and way of dress.

Women and men naturally want to honor their own bodies and the bodies of those around them. No one wants to feel uncomfortable. Some people may not always be in conscious control of their disruptive dress, because it was ingrained in them to dress like that, due to their life experience. Often, if a person is being abused or mistreated, they will express it by wearing negative fashion. Abuse can typically start at a vulnerable young age.

The issue isn't necessarily having to do with women or men appearing attractive. It has to do with using negative sexual force expressed in their fashion for false gain. Clothing can reveal natural beauty and good looks, and that's healthy. However, being sleazy in appearance or overtly power hungry through attire in a sexually domineering way stems from abuse and mistreatment. When life traumas put upon a person are fixed and treated, guaranteed, the person's wardrobe will change. Women and men are no longer beautiful and do not honor themselves when they choose to become a sex object, and it can become a tactic of abusive manipulation. This deprives women and men of their honor. They then become slaves to the artificial, ego-based system of fashion.

There's nothing wrong with women looking beautiful, feminine, and trendy, and men looking attractive, stylish, and cool. Yet, clothing can be offensive by intention and reveal the derogatory characteristics of a tacky, superficial type of apparel. What is wrong is systems of false awareness being forced on society and expressed through dress. It's all about intention, and also about wanting to appear wholesome, creative, and naturally attractive. This approach doesn't promote sex, but promotes beauty and natural good looks.

There's a theory that people dress to attract the opposite sex, or the same sex, depending on one's orientation. But what if we are already taken? Then there's no need to lure anyone. No one wants to feel frumpy and unattractive, however. People genuinely want to feel attracted to themselves and this is done through dressing, for the most part. Fashion is not about sexuality; it is more about expressing creativity and feeling comfortable in one's body. Fashion is about protecting the spirit, and attracting oneself to the spirit within.

Sex sells in fashion because it is part of life. Without sex there's no procreation. The genital area is associated with the root chakra. A person's deep connection with the root chakra, the sexual center, cords people physically to the earth plane, and it is used as a mode of survival. Fashion is definitely a survival-based need. This mode of survival can be expressed through fashion and style in a fear-driven way. Fashion then becomes a source of exploitation.

The root chakra exploited by explicit sexuality expressed in dress degrades the fashion scene, no matter the fashion culture or type of fashion style. Instead of dressing to feel attractive to oneself, people want to attract and pursue others by their way of dress. So, clothing can be performed to take control over other people's root chakra—the groin area, a person's life-force—in a dominating way. It invades personal space and becomes a boundary issue.

Mental and physical abuse occurs when fashion is deliberately used to display vulgarity.

Offensive sexuality in fashion can be liberated when the authenticity and purification of healthy fashion, via natural beauty and attractiveness, overrides the exploitation of fear-driven fashion based on sexual desire, or sex drive. Sexuality in fashion that is amplified from fear of not surviving, and fashion that is ungrounded and low vibration brings people down.

We have a responsibility to evaluate unhealthy fashion, to push modes of dress into transcendence. This will reinforce greater ethical values, and replenish a depleted mental function that's caused by negative fashion appearance. There's deviance in fashion when fashion is in pursuit of expressing sexuality in an exploitative way. Sexually explicit clothing is a revulsion and a perversion to the senses on all fronts.

Attractiveness is not a fault; it is, however, when negatively sexualized. Attraction, in a spiritual sense, acts to protect the body as a sacred temple. Being attractive can be made wholesome and makes everyone, including oneself, feel safe and comfortable. Naturally attractive beauty creates a protection barrier from unnatural beauty.

Fashion can be a tool to look and feel attractive naturally, and not artificially and unnaturally. Unnatural beauty serves negative thinking. The misuse of fashion adornment keeps fashion low. Fashion is about protecting the mind, body, and spirit. Ultimately, a healthy mind, body, and spirit yields a fashion type which will not allow falsehoods or multiple perversions of the senses to enter one's force-field.

No one can look like a sex object if they want to be a holy person of faith and of goodwill. This doesn't mean everyone needs to wear a robe and become a priest, unless that's their path. Fashion that is therapeutic with shielding properties will disperse a harmonic energy that negates any distortion of the body and mind. This can come in many forms in design; and it all depends on intent.

When fashion exploits, fashion cannot be easily recognized as a major self-curing treatment. The discomfort of exploitative clothing alters the senses. This directly applies to the absence of freedom, keeping fashion ineffective, health-wise. Exploitative clothing then resorts to the non-actualization of self, creating discord.

As we enter a new age of great spiritual awakening, we naturally need to confront the issue of sacrificial clothing that serves others, serves things, serves a regime, but no longer serves self. Healthy clothing is aimed at dressing for the self and for protection, and eliminates the lack of boundaries in fashion put upon the wearer and viewer.

Self-objectification found in fashion

Self-objectification is a concern in the fashion industry. Self-objectification is when people view others and themselves as objects for use and not as human beings. Fashion is about selling clothing, not selling the soul. If one sells out to the corrupt part of fashion, it will lead them into a world of mistreatment and dishonor.

Almost everyone has experienced dissociation by wearing

sacrificial dress. Whether voluntarily or involuntarily, we may have felt like an advertisement or a piece of flesh. It doesn't matter if an outfit is revealing or if it's completely covering the body from head to toe, self-objectification expressed in apparel is sacrificial clothing and it comes in many forms.

Self-objectification in fashion can affect a person's mindset. It can create conflicts that instill a threat against others and self. Self-objectification can be cured when the body is dressed in a personally sacred way. The body is a temple and needs to be treated as such. Being gentle to oneself through dress awakens the protective forces of clothing. It will give people a sense of strength and boundaries in oneself.

When clothing is used to objectify the body, it creates an impure body modification. The fashion itself becomes the object, not just the person, because of the way it is used. The modification deliberately attempts to convert the body in a way that diminishes the purpose of fashion for health, and is a symbol of collective defeat. Self-objectification is occurring in every country. It is a violation and form of violence to others, but more so to self.

In all manners of respect, I make no biased approach towards any silhouette from any culture. In terms of the currents of fashion as a whole, all countries have strengths and weaknesses in the name of fashion. But I am going to be using Muslim attire, mostly women's Muslim attire, as an example of self-objectification, because their dress style is a very obvious example of self-objectification in fashion. It's not simply body-revealing apparel, or overtly sexualized apparel that makes a man or woman self-objectified. Objectification in fashion dehumanizes and denies the qualities and character of the objectified person.

The government-regulated clothing of Muslims can be used as an example of self-objectification through dress. I am not confronting their dress in a general way, but in reference to the topic of self-objectification. I am using the Muslim hijab and long dress/tunic as a symbol to represent many other styles and silhouettes that can become, and can appear to be, self-objectified.

Not all Muslim dress relates to self-objectification, and there are subcultures within the Islamic countries and surrounding countries with clothing exceptions, in terms of the strictness and formality of their standard silhouette. The Muslims' formal, law-enforced attire can be found among many other cultures. Their silhouette is not a classic; it is more a traditional costume, because their dress style has not been updated enough over time to keep it fresh, in the name of fashion.

The Muslim people are presumed to call their dress "modest attire." This may create ideas that directly insinuate other styles are immodest, when they are not. For example, if Muslim women have to hide their body, it can create an issue for the rest of the world, and for the people that do not hide their body in their clothes. The body is hidden in such a way that the silhouette tends to give people the idea that if we don't dress in this style, we are not good.

The hyper-clothed body is a message against the body being exposed, and could lead to the defense that the Muslim uniform is better and a less-clothed body is impure. Bear in mind, as we live in a still-sexist environment, women and men are still vulnerable wearing a cloaked dress style. It's because of the heritage behind men and especially women being viewed as objects.

Many Muslim women, for instance, are covered from head to toe, wearing a dress with only her eyes or face visible. This, in some respects, might be an unnatural type of dress. Because it is worn as a uniform, and it can be interpreted as an attempt to serve humans versus serving a higher faith. One reason why this is so is because hiding the face dismisses the celebration of the human body and face to some extent. Furthermore, it can create needless social pressures and potential grievances that hinder self-expression.

Wearing a burqa or hijab—a veil covering the head and face—can make the wearer seem unapproachable, especially when you can only detect them by their eyes. It can further indicate that they are in hiding, and it can be fear-based. It makes it difficult to decipher their expression, remember them, or engage with them. There is also the question of intention behind this type of dress that can be speculated about, because it can prove to express a seductive mysteriousness. The headscarf used in a religious uniform can also be seen as a cover-up of identity. It's a program that covers up people's form of communicating through fashion. It makes it difficult to understand what a person is about. It creates a lack of fashion communication.

Some families demand that the standard dress and hijab be worn. In other instances, wearing it as a free choice could symbolize one's conviction to God. Yet in many parts of the world it is highly discouraged to wear a hat or head covering on certain occasions; it is considered impolite. It is a matter of context and custom, but when a hat is taken off, and the head bows down, it's considered a sign of respect. Overall, the hijab, in many respects, can seem to be a self-righteous form of dress, making it appear as though the wearers have initiated their own ego-based God-attainment, rather than initiating self-surrender to the Almighty Great Spirit.

Muslim dress widely pronounces itself as a tribute to religion and government. Their costume/uniform may be a reflection of laws, economic issues, and political conflict. Many cultures around the world who have a custom uniform may be using it as a way to exploit a lower vibration on Earth. This goes beyond typical traditional silhouettes that are cultural.

In certain areas like Aceh Province, Indonesia, and Iran,

it is the law to wear a hijab. The hijab is the head covering many Muslim women wear. It can be healthy when the style represents modesty. However, their government instructs people to wear this specific fashion style. This rule and law governing the expression of the body may not be a solution for any problem, but may instead result in power and control over humans.

Everyone needs to rise up on the planet. Underdeveloped as well as developed cultures embracing the laws of traditional dress are creating sacrificial requirements that obey man, not spirit, thus going against the evolution of the planet. The apparel industry has been tampered with, so, it can be used as a tool to oppose and separate people and societies.

The Muslim uniform may also not be healthy, in some cases, when everyone is made to look exactly the same. It goes past traditional dress when people are forced to wear a specific look. This can take away feelings of protection of self, and force a person to surrender to the false powers that be.

Muslim men's and women's long dresses/tunics can suggest superiority and royalty relating to religious sentiment. These costume rituals have been developed to work for hierarchical, political schemes which do not match up to the advanced mentality of universal fashion. It's as if clothing is working as a uniform for a governmental operation, and not working for the self.

There's a difference between ceremonial/spiritual dress versus religious, traditional uniforms that make a declaration or revolt against change: fashion evolution. Ceremonial dress like the robe and tunic is celebrated for its property of spiritual resurrection; however, some cultures may exploit the power of spirituality found in the robe and tunic when clothing is turned into a religion and law. For people who want to dress in robes, what makes the difference is if it's done in a healthy, spiritual way. Deliberate ways of dress endured by a whole community in a totalitarian manner may not simply be for a higher power.

It's not necessarily the silhouette, but the wearing of the hijab, robe and tunic as part of a law which halts ideas of spiritual transcendence in fashion. When attire performs as a narrow, government-controlled activity, these fashion laws may be an expression of accrued aggression and outdated conflicts in many uniform-laden regions of the world.

Updating traditional dress for mental health
The Muslim uniform, when it becomes dated, stagnant fashion, in this context, it is not a representation of health. An activity that can be prevented and uplift the Muslim uniform is simply by style variation. This is not about Westernizing fashion, because Westernized fashion needs a lot of help too. It's about universalizing fashion to the degree that we can come to a fashion agreement, speak a similar fashion language, and break down the barriers and conflicts made apparent in fashion. Fashion is a major proponent of either segregation or communion, it needs to speak to many people. Some uniform types create a lack of fashion fluency within many cultures around the world.

Dated fashion can be a sign of old-world thinking. While all this modern fashion has been taking place, traditional dress is managing to say "no" to evolution. Tradition will always remain; fashion laws cannot. Fashion used as a tool to embrace the body, not conform it, is a solution to the growing needs of advancing all of society.

Several different populations following uniform agendas causes mind/body inefficiency. This is creating a malfunction stemmed partly from pride, partly from suppression, and partly for control and power. As long as the uniform is in place, things stay the same. Traditional designs can still be a part of fashion but the innovations of creativity reflected in fashion are to be celebrated for personal and planetary growth.

If cultures want to perceive the body as if it is in need of being hidden, there are lots of modern fashion silhouettes and designs they can embrace and it will still allow their styles and looks to be updated. It's the custom dress that pushes the spirit away to the point where there is deep suppression, and an enclosure of self-identity. Self-identity needs to be expressed for life fulfillment. In reality, many uniforms can disenchant, and sadness and grief from this becomes a burden. Clothing for experimental use should be everyone's right.

Many cultures who wear a uniform are suppressing fashion, not just providing traditional, sentimental aspects of it. It becomes a dated costume too. The silhouette can stay, the colors even, but the attitude behind their way of dress is not religious or spiritual or current if it is in part brought about by laws and used as a negative way to control freedom of speech. It's not a matter of introducing other forms of attire. Women can wear a dress and hijab and it can become modern. However, it's a matter of breaking or stopping laws that prevent the liberation of fashion evolution within all cultures.

When customs of dress conform to laws, and remain stuck as objective materials that fuel the past, we stay in the past. Updating and integrating universal fashion of all cultures around the world will instill further transformation of more contemporary looks. Modern fashion liberates the human being.

Customs will be pushed aside when the influence of modern fashion infiltrates into all runway show collections, shops and streetwear. Modern fashion is found in ready-to-wear shows, where story, theme, and collective forces of inspiration are shared, to keep life interesting. Fashion shows add fuel to the fire when things get low. The power of fashion is needed via fashion shows. The fashion themes in fashion shows and fashion collections need to be produced to introduce new modes of creation. Fashion shows presented twice or more a year give people hope for a future of new ideas. Cultures susceptible to government regulations of dress need to be influenced by new stories, new artistic innovations, new ways of thinking.

All in all, many uniforms are an example of protesting against natural fashion cycles, and can be viewed as anti-fashion, bringing an uninviting aesthetic to the public at large. They are going against current fashion that is made up as a major conductor of trends, holistic style cycles, and fashion evolution. Fashion is part of the performance of everyday life.

Trends are valuable because they become personal milestones for the industry and the wardrobe.

Additionally, there's an innate motive to present seasonal trends contributing to, and in reflection of, an ever-evolving planet. It is the natural rhythms of life that are the most important influence on fashion. Fashion-trend milestones mark periods in history and represent the times. These styles evolve, move, and grow along with the planet's natural evolution. Universal fashion acts as a gateway to remove the limitations of suppressed fashion within all cultures.

Anti-fashion: fashion that goes against the human

When I speak about anti-fashion, I am not talking about the style genres: punk rocker, or grunge. Many style genres do promote some evil-influenced fashion. They suppress a person's life-force and encourage death energy. A few clothing features — spiky edges, fetish, and clothing that looks like a mutated form of another species — are clear examples of spiritless, anti-fashion. Some of the designs that are associated with these genres may be anti-fashion, but anti-fashion is what it sounds like: fashion that goes against the human. Fashion that lacks a spiritual force. Anti-fashion garments also imply a lack of spirited connection to the wearer and a lack of authenticity.

Anti-fashion can throw off the wearer and observer psychologically and physically. It can be expressed as an energetic attack, creating a low, negative vibration. Clothing may not make someone sick to their stomach, but in reality, it can, whether it is subtle or obvious. This happens from either fabric based, to the art of design placement, to the measurement of life-producing chi energy flowing through a design, and so on.

Fashion rebelling against natural, collective trends is anti-fashion. Where cultural community identities are dressing for segregation, this can bankrupt the soul; this is anti-fashion. Clothing cannot be a therapeutic treatment when anti-fashion prevents people from being their true self. This disconnection disables power, keeping fashion from what it can truly be and become.

Negative vibrations can come from symbols like the crossbone, skull, hex symbol, spikes, weaponry, death symbols, and so on. Fashion exploitation occurs when these fashion symbols and beauty rituals from traditional cultures are inappropriately used and created with wrong intent. Death reaper-like fashion, like hollowed-out skeletons with hex symbols, has a cold demeanor and can be a representation of evil. Fashion that transmutes people into morbid creatures is dehumanizing.

The use of crossbones, skeletons, and bones as decoration still goes on today. It exploits animals depending on its arrangement displayed on the body. Native Americans used animal bones appropriately. Tribal people have worn animal bones, teeth, and even blood under their eyes as makeup. These are customs and rites belonging to their personal lifestyle.

Rites can be identified and then used and distorted in an unfamiliar way by modern society. There's really no way to understand or evaluate rites based upon no direct experience.

Their lifestyle and life practice is different. Yet evil-influenced fashion can still be evil, even by the tribes themselves, as some are cultish and use satanic practice.

The death symbol incorporated in fashion apparel and accessories is a custom for some cultures. Some of these cultures perceive death differently and it is not a morbid expression. Cultural symbols, if used positively, can add value to a fashion design, and can perform as part of an initiation, and be an important feature of a look. But cultural symbols exploited and turned for the worse are negatively channeled in various detrimental ways. They misalign with nature and exploit culture. Death symbol fashion is acceptable only until this evil-influenced type of dress is revealed as offensive to others and the environment.

Demonizing death becomes a setback. Seeing death as a primordial symbol of afterlife is one thing. For example, Mexico's traditional holiday, the Day of the Dead, is celebrated. It doesn't deliver evil sentiment. Using symbols wrongfully, however, yields very hideous ramifications, whether it be conscious or unconscious. Some fashions cross the line when they are evil-influenced. It's not always the designer's fault. It can stem from a collective attitude, from the subconscious of a negative society.

Soulless fashion stems from evil-influenced, satanic practice. Evil-influenced satanic practice is a manipulation of energy that comes from a false, artificial, evil force. The intent and impression behind many negative symbols contribute to satanic practices. Demons, negative entities, and other types of soulless non-beings who do not have internal energy reserves and resources of energy tend to parasite off of another's light force, and extract power from external forces and people, manipulating and distorting energy. This is not spiritual or ethical, and doesn't extend itself to a practice of working with divine consciousness.

There is a negative factor to evil-influenced, spiritless fashion. In extreme ways, it can represent a "lost soul" condition. Fashion can channel dark spirits to a certain degree. Anti-fashion can also be a contributing factor of soul possession. Evil-influenced fashion cannot protect the spirit of life.

When evil is practiced in fashion there's an eerie feeling, and some of the fashion industry participates. There is pride, ego, and false awareness involved when fashion is created for the sake of onlookers to be in awe of it. In many cases, clothing can enable satanic worship and false power. This can strike chords of negativity that deflate the mood and weaken a person's spirit.

Fashion and evil combined is not good, and negative interferences occur. People are naturally intuitive and are cautious about this. To be in a realm of higher consciousness, fashion consumers and fashion professionals need to protect themselves, because fashion is naturally a channel and can evoke either high or low vibrations.

The negative influences of anti-fashion

Any inclination to view clothes as frivolity lies within the means of disconnection to self, and disconnection with the Earth and Universe. Clothing used as a guide, a directional tool, is an active pursuit of surrendering. Healthy fashion eliminates controlling activities presented in wrongful dress. Wrongful dress is a means of lack, an emptiness, it feels and looks controlled. It is a form of suppression and is an additional contribution to the artificial toxicities of the world. It defines something no one genuinely wants to be a part of or represent. It only fuels the desire of a perpetual cycle of negative habitual repetition of anti-fashion. This goes against the harmonic cyclical course of healthy fashion which can be positively used as an instrument for transcendence.

Anti-fashion limits fashion perspectives and is a nuisance in its behaviors and actions that go against humanity. As an example, an outfit that looks great but feels uncomfortable is a quick fix, creating static and stagnant energy. When humans gravitate towards temporary fashion solutions, these clothes will create a perpetual, habitual feeling of control and discomfort. Additionally, the depressive forces of evil remove the spiritual hygiene of fashion for self-care. It is true, fashion can express different forms of disease and negative symptoms, if we look closely.

Many times, there can be a disconnect between a person and some of the looks they wear. Many wardrobes often have a mix of spiritual fashion and spiritless fashion. For example, when a person isn't feeling completely alive or awake, we can put on clothing that lacks identity, and it can make us feel even more somber, and irritated. There can be a consistent or even redundant intrusion of certain outfits that do not provide levels of ease. This destabilizes and disrupts the day, and uproots the days when a look flawlessly agrees with us. As our connection to clothing improves, tendencies to not wear anti-fashion improve.

There will always be at least a little negativity in life, and this negativity is sometimes expressed in fashion design and style. When negativity exceeds to a point where it's offensive and obtrusive, it falls into ego-based cycles of wrong intent. It also creates a lack of boundary.

The saying that we have to take the good with the bad is not entirely true. We can transmute negativity much more than what we are currently transmuting as a collective society on this planet.

Fashion that is negative and turns punishing when expressed outward on another or on oneself shouldn't be acceptable. This abusive mistreatment is immoral and ultimately goes beyond the duality of positive and negative. Fashion should practice the yin and yang concept, not the good versus bad concept. There is a difference between yin and yang, and good versus evil. Many fashions express the good and evil. However, the yin and yang concept is an expression of night and day, or sun and moon, not good and bad. The truth of the matter is, small amounts of negativity can exist, but evil cannot. Polarity and duality in fashion need to be limited.

The yin/yang, masculine/feminine elements can be the basis of symbolism in fashion to override the overindulgence of apparel treated to "possess" oneself or others via a negative force. Some fashion designs exist in a negative vibration if the person's interests are of ill intent. It's evil, if evil intent is involved. We need more yin and yang concepts in fashion to override the interest of having to celebrate good versus bad. The bad shouldn't even be acknowledged, it's just feeding the fire of more negatively-influenced fashion.

Fashion and existentialism

Fashion can become moderately existential in different stages of life. There are multiple perceptions registered between fashion, humans, and existentialism. The root of existentialism is sometimes formed by an internal human condition that's based on external conditions. So, it's when people are forced to internalize based on external conditions. This fashion existentialist point of view provokes contemplation during trying times, thus inhibiting a fashion perception turned conscious.

Fashion existentialism can prove to be, at times, an expulsion of spirit. Existentialism often involves purgatory-like regimes that play a role in habitual suffering from the expulsion of spirit. However, it also is a place of purging and releasing, which persists to evolve a person's soul.

There are moments when there is a sense of emptiness towards the ways of dress. This is partly created from a ready-made portrait of fashion's conditional standards placed upon society, which offers an overly devalued testament of clothing's true meaning and purpose.

There are two distinct forms of existentialism in conjunction with fashion. One form is the existential fashion/human relationship; clothing being a reflection and connection within an existential existence. Developing a deep relationship with clothing extends itself as an opportunity to really understand the relationship with the external. Existentialism in fashion also makes people aware that clothing is not always a reflection of a person.

The other form of fashion existentialism is fashion itself portraying and expressing existentialism. This could lead to purgatory-like fashions that feel like sacrificial imprisonment. Other times when fashion is made as a safe zone creating mental strength and awareness, this is when clothing is a sanctuary.

Fashion existentialism usually creates experiences and evokes feelings that can lead to resurrection. The clothing itself is holy, and is a personal experience of faith expressing itself through fashion. This is when fashion can create spiritual breakthroughs for a person. This is brought forth through a very spiritual persistence of fashion evidently providing, spiritually. What transpires is that in order to have a healthy relationship with fashion, we have to honor our experience, and our participation in wardrobe and outfit selections, as it is partially an embodiment of spiritual presence and health.

PART 3

PLANT-BASED FABRICS AND DYES

Chapter 8

The 36 Plant-based Fashion Fabrics for the Present and Future

A plant-based fabric future

Given the increasing limitations and health setbacks that synthetic fabrics provide, plant-based fabrics are much more of an asset and a future prevalent. Plant-based fabrics will help resist disease and support health as they are medicinal and therapeutic. They will help human health, the economy, social balance, global balance, and the environment.

Scientists claim there are about 391,000 plant species worldwide, and many plant species and plants are still to be discovered. Between 550 and 700 different plants were used in the production of textiles in the Southwest of America alone. Important plants that were historically produced into textiles need to be brought back into production, and in further pursuit of their textile development.

The modern world is limited to only a handful of plant-based fabric types. Fabrics made from a variety of plants offer more support to the wearer versus wearing fabrics made from only a couple of different plants. Wearing a variety of colored dyes and fabric types can be likened to eating a rainbow-like assortment of foods with their varying nutritional properties.

A few top plant-based fabrics that are currently accessible for the mass market:

- cotton
- hemp
- linen
- ramie

- nettle
- bamboo (natural)
- abaca
- kapok
- lyocell

A few top minor fabrics that are currently accessible for the niche market, and have great potential to be produced for mass scale:

- paper fiber (paper yarn)
- seacell
- cactus silk
- sasawashi
- lotus
- pina

In addition to these 15 fabrics you will find the complete inspiring collection of 36 exceptional plant-based fabrics below. All of them are to be on the lookout for, and need to be increased in production for the present and future time.

About the 36 plant-based fashion fabrics and their detailed descriptions

A detailed description of 36 plant-based fabrics is included here. Decriptions of the fabrics' properties, use, function, performance, and their aesthetic variations are included. It's a fabric archive and a useful tool. It can be used for sourcing fabrics, shopping, research, reference, and simply for the benefit of identifying the plant-based fabrics of the future. It can also be an inspirational resource, in order to drive their development and infiltrate them into the fashion industry markets.

These plant-based fabric varieties are a top choice for

the future of the fashion and textile industry. Imagine the possibilities of cotton, hemp, linen, nettle, ramie, bamboo, abaca, banana, pina, cactus silk, coir, and more. The range of "plant-tech" fabrics is numerous and ever-evolving.

Each of the 36 fabrics listed contain the following detailed descriptions and their content/information:

Fabric features: What the plant-fiber/fabric is about.

Fiber characteristics: Specific traits and textile performance properties of the fabric.

Texture: What the fabric looks and feels like.

Therapeutic properties: The fabric's health properties and therapeutic benefits.

Sustainability: What makes the fabric eco and sustainable.

History: Where the fabric originated from, and the history of the fabric.

Availability: The fabric's measured availability; they're either high availability, moderate availability, minor availability, or vast potential.

About the "Availability" fabric description

The fabrics listed have an "availability" description that indicates the quantity of these plant fibers that are currently being produced: "High availability," "Moderate availability," or "Minor availability" of the fabric. Not all 36 fabrics listed are currently in production. So, included are fabrics with "Vast potential." "Vast potential" fabrics are proven to be worthy of industrial production but aren't in production, or are currently being produced very minimally. All have been successfully tested and studied, or have been made into a fabric at one point, however.

Some fabrics included have already been produced in ancient times or more recently in history, but they are no longer being produced on a minor or major scale. But they have vast potential for future use. While only a handful of plant-based fabric varieties are dominating the current industry, listed are extensive, biodiverse plant fiber varieties, all capable of being produced in bulk.

About the "Therapeutic properties" fabric description

The "therapeutic property" description is specific to the health benefits these plants provide in their whole form, and often when they are ingested. I do not make claims that these therapeutic properties of the plant listed will extend themselves in the plants' fabric form. The therapeutic properties listed are not all necessarily going to occur when the plant fibers are in textile form. Further studies are needed to prove these therapeutic properties of the plant work for the body in its textile form.

The therapeutic properties of the fabrics listed are in terms of their healing capabilities in their general use. They are included to reveal the healing powers of these plants. For example, kudzu root, taken as an herb, comes in the form of a powder and is ingested to treat muscle pain, gastritis and injury. Kudzu fabric may also induce these same health benefits when the plant fiber is worn topically.

The therapeutic properties of the plant fibers listed are not all scientifically proven, yet these plant-based fabrics have true healing potential for their use as a topical treatment. For example, bamboo, by its texture and appearance, is naturally therapeutic. The calming and soothing effects of bamboo fabric support mental health.

The therapeutic properties of these plant fibers can also be carried over through their energetic composition, just like the red and green colored towels Hanna Kroeger asked her patients to cover themselves in overnight for their healing benefits. It's this unusual concept that the frequency of these colors creates a healing effect, just the same as these plant fabrics' frequency can perform that way when they are worn.

These plant fibers will perform medically for the wearer in multiple ways. Keep in mind, healthy fashion is not just about the plant fibers. Plant-based fabrics' treatments, fabric finishes, fabric dye, and laundry detergents are all going to play a role and give additional health and healing benefits for the mind, body and spirit.

The six mutual health benefits of the 36 plant-based fabric varieties

There are six standard therapeutic/health properties listed below that each of the 36 plant-based fabrics have. I am going to list them here because they are all mutually effective in every plant fabric. They are not included under every fabric listed, because it would be redundant for you to read them 36 different times.

The six standard, therapeutic/health properties prominent in each plant fiber:

- **Supports oxygen levels:** Plant fabrics have a breathability property that keeps the skin healthy. They promote and produce oxygen within the body.
- **Stimulates and improves blood flow and circulation:** Plant fabrics have ergonomic surface textures. Down to their cellular level, they have the ability to soothe, invigorate, and revitalize the skin, and in effect, it gives the skin a subtle massage that soothes and protects the nerves.
- **Chemical composition-balanced:** Plant-based fabrics have a chemical composition that supports the chemical makeup of the body. This helps the body resonate in one's own skin comfortably. When worn, they give a

beneficial skin and body treatment.

- **Ergonomic:** Plant-based fibers are naturally ergonomic, from the fiber's cellular level up to the point of their final yarn or fabric. Ergonomic fabrics adapt to the body on an intuitive and physiological level.
- **Hypoallergenic/hygienic:** Plant-based fabrics are hypoallergenic, for the most sensitive types of skin. They are clean fabrics that keep us feeling fresh.
- **Anti-stress:** Studies prove that when people go out into nature, stress reduction results. Wearing "nature" on the body can instantly provide a plant/human connection that reduces stress.

The essential, standard, sustainability benefits of wearing and producing plant fibers that are mutual to all 36 plant-based fabrics

There are also several standard sustainability properties listed below that each of the 36 plant-based fibers have. I am going to list them here because they are all mutually effective in every plant fabric.

The mutual sustainability properties of all 36 plant fibers: Eco-friendly, biodegradable, renewable, self-sustaining, a natural wasted resource, supports biodiversity, restorative sustainable, recyclable, they can be blended with other plant fibers.

The 36 plant-based fashion fabrics

Please note: Not all properties and characteristics are listed under each fabric. This is a sample description of each fabric, which includes some of their major characteristics and information.

Not every plant fabric is listed but several of the most

sought-after and promising are.

ABACA
Fabric features: Abaca is a bast/stem and leaf fiber from the banana family Musaceae. It is also named banana hemp, and manila hemp. It is a non-fruit bearing herbaceous flowering plant. It's a great fabric for shirting, water-resistant outerwear, raincoats, and accessories. An abaca paper yarn has been developed for sweaters and other knitwear. Abaca fiber has also been developed and produced into durable denim fabric.

Fiber characteristics: Breathable, water-repellent, moisture-wicking, resilient, high tensile strength, durable, flexible, antibacterial, deodorizing, grease-repellent, fire-resistant, emits heat.

Texture: Abaca fabric has a lustrous sheen. It's soft, silky, similar to organza silk, and it can be as durable as denim.

Therapeutic properties: It has natural, protective properties. It strengthens bones and tissues, as it is used as a biocomposite.

Sustainability: Self-sustaining, and minimizes soil erosion.

History: Abaca is native to the Philippine Islands, the indigenous Higaonon tribe of Mindanao, Indonesia, Costa Rica, and Ecuador. It has been historically used for kimonos, saris, and tablecloths.

Availability: Moderate availability.

AGAVE, *americana l.*
Fabric features: Agave is a cellulosic leaf fiber, and a long vegetable fiber. It is a cactus-like plant, also named maguey, the century plant, and American aloe. There are about 300 species of agave. Various kinds of the agave cactus can be turned into fabrics. Agave fabric is typically used in accessories and embroidery; however,

new testing is being done to process it into an apparel fabric.

Fiber characteristics: Flexibility, high tensile strength, high elasticity. It's hydrophilic, it absorbs water and releases it faster than cotton and wool.

Texture: Agave fabric varieties range from coarse to silk-like and lustrous.

Therapeutic properties: In Aztec tradition, the goddess Mayheul was recognized as the personification of the maguey plant. The plant symbolizes long life, health, dancing, and fertility.

Sustainability: Rapidly renewable, self-sustaining. When its leaves are cut and pruned, new leaves grow, keeping the plant alive for much longer.

History: Agave is native to Mexico, Arizona, Central America, and originates from Europe, Guatemala, Africa, and the Far East. Agave fiber has been made into products since the time of the Aztec civilization.

Availability: Minor availability. Vast potential (for apparel).

ALOE VERA

Fabric features: Aloe vera is a cellulosic leaf fiber. It's known as the "lily of the desert." Additionally, the inner gel of the aloe plant is used in the fabric treatments and fiber infusions of cosmetic apparel.

Fiber characteristics: Breathability, repels moisture, high tensile strength, low extensibility, antibacterial, thermal-balanced.

Texture: Soft, durable, similar to bamboo fabric.

Therapeutic properties: It's known as the "plant of immortality" and for its medicinal effects. It is skin-softening, and traditionally used as a nourishing skin treatment.

Sustainability: A natural food by-product, highly

renewable.

History: Aloe vera is native to the Arabian Peninsula, and cultivated in Africa and India.

Availability: Minor availability. Vast potential.

ALOE VERA CACTUS, SAHARAN

Fabric features: The Saharan aloe vera cactus is a genus of monocots, found in the sub-family of agavoideae. It is a silk alternative, called "vegetable sylk," or "sabra silk."

Fiber characteristics: Strength, durability, high elasticity, wrinkle-resistant.

Texture: It has a soft, silky, metallic sheen. Some fabric types are duller in appearance.

Therapeutic properties: They have a plethora of medicinal uses, and the cactus can also be made into therapeutic cactus flower essences.

Sustainability: Highly renewable, fast-growing, a natural waste food industry by-product.

History: The Saharan aloe vera plant is popularly grown in the Sahara Desert, and is found and made prominently in Morocco and Spain. It is commonly used in decorative motifs, home goods, accessories, jackets, and other apparel. The Aztec people used to make rope and twine out of it.

Availability: Minor availability. Vast potential.

BAMBOO

Fabric features: Bamboo belongs to the grass family Poaceae. Natural bamboo is an important plant for apparel use. There's a difference between natural bamboo fabric and viscose bamboo fabric. Natural bamboo, also named bamboo linen, or original bamboo, is processed mechanically. Bamboo viscose is chemically processed.

We shouldn't eliminate bamboo because of the

"viscose" type processing. There are natural bamboo fabrics that do not use this processing. Also, there is a bamboo lyocell, a chemical process made with less toxic chemicals. This is much preferred over the viscose process.

Tests by the Japanese Textile Inspection Association revealed a 70% death rate of bacteria on bamboo fabric. This is caused by the natural, antibacteria bio-agent, "bamboo kun," which is a part of the bamboo cellulose.

Fiber characteristics: Breathability, ventilation, moisture absorption, moisture vapor transmission, wicking, tensile strength, elasticity, temperature balance, cooling and warming, antimicrobial, antibacterial, antifungal, odor-resistant, deodorization, antistatic, wrinkle-resistant.

Texture: Luster, drape, softness, and smoothness.

Therapeutic properties: It's used in traditional Asian medicine. Bamboo fabric has a soothing and calming tactility. The plant has anti-aging health benefits for hair, skin, and nails, and is a collagen booster. Bamboo is used as a material to prevent damage from earthquakes. The material is designed to "dance" with the earthquake.

Sustainability: A highly renewable plant, grows rapidly, improves soil, and produces 35% more oxygen than trees. It's one of the fastest-growing grasses.

History: Bamboo is an ancient medicine in Ayurveda, and Chinese acupuncture. Bamboo is revered as a mystical plant, as it's popularly named: "Lucky bamboo." It's a symbol of strength.

Availability: Moderate availability (bamboo linen). Moderate availability (bamboo lyocell).

BANANA

Fabric features: Banana fabric is made from the stalk and leaf of the fruit-bearing tree. Banana fabric is a plant "sylk" alternative. It produces both coarse and fine fibers. A banana fiber separator machine has been developed in India by Tiruchirappalli Regional Engineering College, Science and Technology Entrepreneurs Park.

Fiber characteristics: Breathable, moisture absorption, high-moisture and absorption release, wicking, tensile strength, fire-resistant, heat-resistant.

Texture: Silky sheen, soft, supple, a likeness to hemp and bamboo.

Therapeutic properties: The banana plant's leaf and stem contain various curative properties.

Sustainability: Banana stems, stalks, and leaves are a by-product of the food industry, making this fiber a natural waste food industry by-product. One billion tons of banana stems are wasted each year.

History: Banana fabric has been cultivated in Japanese and Southeast Asian cultures since the thirteenth century. Deities and gods in ancient times were represented by material symbols, such as banana. Banana fabric replaced zari and weaving motifs due to the banana fibers' gold-like appearance and color. In Nepal, they used the pulp of banana bark and spun it into yarn.

Availability: Minor availability. Vast potential.

CATTAIL, *typha latifolia*

Fabric features: Cattails come from the family of Typhaceae. Found in the wetlands, the cattail is an herbaceous perennial plant. Its short, fluffy fibers are found in the cylindrical flower (seedpods) of the cattail plant. Its seedpod is filled with fibers which can be used as an insulating material. It is a plant-down alternative for thermal apparel, as a padding material, and it can made into fabric.

Cattail fluff maintains buoyancy after 100 hours of submersion. Its stalk/leaf can also be used as a fiber source for textiles. The fiber is 60–80% cellulose, which yields great potential to be produced as a fabric.

Fiber characteristics: Moisture regain, mold-resistant, insulating, thermal, fire-resistant, a highly prolific crenulated structure.

Texture: Its seedpod fluff is soft and buoyant. Its leaf/stalk fibers have similar behaviors and appearance to cotton and linen.

Therapeutic properties: Its flotation-like buoyancy and levitation effect is therapeutic. It was formerly used as a wound dressing. It is a healing plant for illness, and is purifying.

Sustainability: Using cattails in textiles will contribute to environmental protection. The aquatic weed is a natural, wasted resource, and a soil regenerator. A study of the fiber's efficiency, quality, and characterization of cattail fibers for textile applications stated that "Their growth rate is enormous."

History: Cattails are located in North America, the Great Lakes, the Everglades, and in the temperate and colder regions of the Northern and Southern hemispheres. Native Americans used it as a moccasin lining.

Availability: Vast potential.

CEDAR BARK

Fabric features: Cedar bark can be felted, braided, crocheted, and so on. The "bark cloth" can be used for accessories. It can also be used as a medicinal dye. More technology is needed for it to be developed into a fabric.

Fiber characteristics: Breathable, strength, pliable.

Texture: Soft, matte.

Therapeutic properties: In many tribes, cedar is used in plant medicine. Cedar bark is associated with prayer, dreams, healing, and protection. Cedar wood incense is known to clear the energy body of toxins and negative energy.

Sustainability: Renewable, self-sustaining, biodegradable.

History: Cedar bark cloth was used by the indigenous people of the Pacific Northwest, Canada, USA, and made by people of Baganda and Uganda. Historically, the bark cloth was predominantly used.

Availability: Minor availability. Vast potential.

COCONUT

Fabric features: The coconut (coir) fibers are extracted from the coconut husk. Coconut-derived fabrics can perform in a variety of apparel uses such as outerwear and accessories. Typically found in geotextiles, the fibers of coconut husks can be used as insulation materials for cold-weather and outdoor apparel. Coir works well as a fiber blend. The shell of the coconut is popularly used for buttons and trims.

Fiber characteristics: Ventilation, moisture retention, antimicrobial, antibacterial, fast-drying, high resistance, abrasion resistant, thermal, insulating.

Texture: Coarse to fine.

Therapeutic properties: It supports the body ergonomically. Its texture stimulates circulation. It has great potential as a material used in acupressure fashion, and accessories.

Sustainability: A natural waste food industry by-product. Around 50 billion coconuts fall from coconut trees annually. Supports soil erosion.

History: Coconut trees are found in tropical regions, and are popular in India, Sri Lanka, Bangladesh, Thailand, and Nigeria. The Kiribati tribe used coconuts in their armor apparel.

Availability: Minor availability. Vast potential.

CORK, *quercus suber l.*

Fabric features: Cork is a vegan leather harvested from the bark of the oak tree. The bark itself has a honeycomb structure made of many holes, making the cork fabric airy and lightweight. It's made into accessories like jewelry, hats, bags, wallets, watch bands, and shoes. Cork fabric can be used to make raincoats and jackets. It's great for outdoor apparel, and is used as a thermal insulator.

Fiber characteristics: Breathable, hypoallergenic, waterproof, thermoregulating, durable, buoyant, insect-repellent, stain-resistant, fire-resistant, thermal, insulating.

Texture: Supple, soft, flexible.

Therapeutic properties: Oak bark is commonly taken as an herb. It's an antioxidant. It is naturally ergonomic due to its buoyancy. Its flotation property is soothing. It has therapeutic, shock and sound absorption properties.

Sustainability: Cork oak forests help prevent desertification and deforestation. Stripping the bark does not harm the tree, it helps it to naturally grow back. Stripped oak bark trees absorb five times more CO_2.

History: Cork has been used for thousands of years as a flotation device, and for home insulation.

Availability: High availability (for accessories). Minor availability (for apparel).

CORN, HUSK

Fabric features: The husk of the corn is a long, cellulosic fiber from the grass family Poaceae. It is the green, leafy outer layer covering the corn that is to be used for textiles. This textile differs from Ingeo™ corn fiber. Ingeo is not recommended, and the fabric is made from the edible part of corn, its kernels. Corn husk is a relatively unknown fiber resource discovered by scientist Yiqi Yang. Corn husk fiber has more elasticity than most other plant fibers. When blended with other plant fibers, this makes it a suitable, ergonomic addition. It has a higher dye pickup than cotton.

Fiber characteristics: Breathable, high moisture retention, tensile strength, elasticity, pliability.

Texture: It has properties similar to cotton and linen.

Therapeutic properties: Corn husks are used to treat medical conditions, and are most specifically used as a pain reliever.

Sustainability: It's highly renewable, and an agricultural waste by-product. It's the second largest agricultural crop in the world. Corn husks are a natural waste food industry by-product. It needs to be non-GMO.

History: A relatively new fiber, corn husk fabric was developed by textile scientist Yiqi Yang, from the University of Nebraska. He created a patented process that extracts fibers from corn husks, and the fibers are turned into a yarn and fabric. Corn husks are generally used to preserve and wrap food.

Availability: Vast potential.

COTTON

Fabric features: Cotton is a seed fiber that grows in the seed pod or boll. Bt cotton, a GMO cotton seed, is widespread. Organic cotton production is merely 1% on a global scale, and an average of 95% of cotton is genetically modified in India and the US. The need for more organic or non-GMO cotton crops is essential.

Cotton seed fiber absorbs 20% water vapor without feeling wet. It can hold up to 65% of its own weight of water without dripping. It can also absorb moisture from high-humidity environments.

Fiber characteristics: Breathable, hypoallergenic, moisture absorption, quick-drying, tensile strength, antistatic, conducts heat away from the body.

Texture: Soft and smooth.

Therapeutic properties: Soft, soothing. A very calming yet uplifting fabric.

Sustainability: If cotton is genetically modified, it's not sustainable. If it can't be made organic, multiple cotton certification programs offer non-organic options that are highly suitable.

History: In 1793, the cotton gin was invented which created cotton demand. Archeological finds of cotton fabrics have been documented in India and Pakistan in 6000 BC.

Availability: High availability.

HEMP

Fabric features: Hemp is a bast/stem fiber, a great alternative to cotton and linen. Bioplastic, hemp fabric can be made useful for weather proof outerwear and an alternative to petroleum-based polyester fabrics. The fibers can be produced into coarse to fine yarn.

Fiber characteristics: Breathable, moisture-wicking, water absorption (absorbs 20% moisture without feeling damp), thermoregulation, shape retention, tensile strength, antibacterial, mold/mildew-resistant, durability, non-static, conducts heat away from the body, insulating.

Texture: Naturally lustrous, soft.

Therapeutic properties: Hemp oil is often used as an herbal remedy.

Sustainability: It needs little to no chemicals to harvest, it does not need herbicides and fungicides to grow. Highly renewable; a full harvest takes 3–4 months. It needs less water to cultivate as compared to cotton. It also requires less land than cotton and linen to yield the same crop amount. Hemp absorbs more CO_2 than trees.

History: Hemp textiles were initially produced in the 1820s. Hemp originated in Southeast Asia, and was recorded as early as 2800 BC. It spread throughout Europe, Spain, Chile, and North America. In 150 BC, hemp was popular in paper making. Buddhist texts from the second and third century AD were printed on hemp paper.

Availability: High availability.

JUTE, *corchorus olitorius, corchorus capsularis*

Fabric features: Jute is a bast/stem fiber. It is known as the "golden fabric." It's used in accessories like shoes, bags, etc. There is a "woolenized" jute that is good for denim and outerwear. As it is a naturally coarse fiber, the ring spinning textile process can produce a finer yarn. There are two variations: a tough coarse fiber, and a fine fiber. The finest jute fibers can imitate silk and linen. This vegetable sylk alternative can be used for formal apparel, evening wear, and accessories.

Fiber characteristics: Breathable, moisture-wicking, fast-drying, high tenacity, antistatic, sound and heat insulating.

Texture: Soft, shiny, silk-like.

Therapeutic properties: It was traditionally used as medicine by the Egyptians and Indians. The leaf part of the plant is used as an herbal remedy.

Sustainability: It grows without pesticides and fertilizers. It's highly renewable and self-sustaining; 2.47 acres of jute can absorb as much as 15 tons of CO_2 and release 11 tons of oxygen in a matter of 100 days.

History: Jute is found in the major parts of East and West Bengal. India and Bangladesh are its top producers. Jute sylk is commonly used for silk saris.

Availability: High availability. Vast potential (for apparel).

KAPOK

Fabric features: The kapok tree, also named the cotton and ceiba tree, bears fruit pods. Seed hair fibers in the form of a silky fluff are found inside these seedpods. It is also named the bombacaceae tree, the silk cotton tree in Thailand, and kapok in Malaysia and the Philippines.

It's useful as padding/filling material and insulation for garments.

Its cell structure allows it to trap air for insulation. Kapok fiber is a great wool alternative. Kapok keeps afloat 30–35 times its weight, cork only 5 times its weight. Kapok can also be made into a fabric or blended with other fibers. The tree can reach up to 200 feet, and grow up to 13 feet per year.

Fiber characteristics: Breathable, hypoallergenic, moisture-resistant, water-repellent, quick-drying, anti-clumping, shape retention, anti-mold, anti-decay, vermin-resistant, pest-resistant, insulating, thermal.

Texture: It's soft like cotton, and organza silk-like. It's softer and lighter than feather-down.

Therapeutic properties: Several parts of the kapok tree are used as an herbal treatment.

Sustainability: It's naturally grown without chemicals or pesticides, and prevents deforestation.

History: Mt. Everest explorers tested boots successfully designed by SATRA. These boots were made with kapok insulation for its warmth value. These high-altitude climbing boots were a part of the successful conquest in 1953 by the British Everest Expedition. The kapok tree is sacred in Mayan mythology. Mayans believed it stood at the center of the earth. The kapok tree is considered sacred, "With its roots reaching the underworld, and branches holding up the sky," as told by Mayans. It was originally used for mattress stuffing, pillow-stuffing, and life-jackets.

Availability: High availability.

KENAF, *hibiscus cannabinus*

Fabric features: Kenaf is a long bast fiber. 50% of the kenaf stalk is fiber. Kenaf comes from the Malvaceae family. Kenaf is related to okra, cotton and hemp. It has great potential for apparel use.

Fiber characteristics: Natural absorbency, high tensile strength, fire-retardant.

Texture: Soft, lustrous, it resembles linen and hemp.

Therapeutic properties: It is used as a dietary fiber supplement and taken as an herbal remedy.

Sustainability: Fast growing, highly renewable, absorbs more CO_2 than any other plant. Every hectare of crop consumes more than 30–40 tons of carbon dioxide from each growing cycle. It's drought-tolerant, and restores deforestation.

History: Originating in Asia and East Africa, kenaf is a major crop in Asia and Africa, popularly grown in India, USA, Malaysia, Vietnam, and Thailand. It was used by the Ancient Egyptians, and documented from 1000 BC.

Availability: High availability (for home decor). Vast potential (for apparel).

KUDZU

Fabric features: Kudzu fiber is a long bast fiber. It's also named Japanese arrowroot, kudzu-fu or ko-hemp. It's a climbing vine from the pea family, Fabaceae. It's an invasive weed which makes it a great, natural resource for apparel.

Fiber characteristics: Breathable, water-resistant.

Texture: Supple, shiny.

Therapeutic properties: Kudzu root starch is used as an herbal supplement, and contains allantoin, which supports healthy skin.

Sustainability: Highly renewable, grows rapidly, an aggressive weed.

History: Kudzu fiber is native to Asia, and currently grown in the southeastern United States. It's prevalent in Japan. They used to make kudzu cloth in Japan for centuries. According to Chinese mythology, in ancient times there was a saint called Ge-tian-shi. In the region he was called "He-nan-sheng," who taught people how to make clothes and shoes out of twisted kudzu threads.

Availability: Minor availability. Vast potential.

LEMBA, *capitulata, curculigo latifolia*

Fabric features: Lemba, also named daun doyo, is a leaf fiber. Lemba, a wild, wetland grass leaf, was used predominantly in indigenous cultures for textile use.

Fiber characteristics: Absorbent, strong, durable, static-resistant, tenacity, abrasion-resistant.

Therapeutic properties: A Chinese medicinal herb. In Borneo, the leaves were used in magical healing ceremonies.

Texture: Similar to linen.

Sustainability: Fast-growing, self-sustaining.

History: Lemba is found in swampy areas in Asia, Australia, Malaysia, Thailand, and Japan. It was a predominant fiber in ancient times. Indigenous people of Sarawak produced lemba fabric and used it to produce a natural textile dye.

Availability: Vast potential.

LINEN, *linum usitatissimum*

Fabric features: Linen, also named flax, is a bast fiber. There are up to 200 flax varieties. It reduces gamma radiation and is two to three times stronger than cotton. It becomes softer after washing and can hold up to 20% water without feeling damp. The heat conductivity of linen is five times higher than wool.

Linen has cooling properties due to its hollow fibers which circulate air and regulate temperature. It absorbs moisture from the air. Petroleum-based fabrics do not have this moisture-absorbing property, creating electrical static and making skin dry.

Fabric characteristics: Breathable, hypoallergenic, ventilation, air permeability, thermoregulation, warming, cooling, hygroscopic (absorbs moisture without feeling damp), moisture-wicking, fast-drying, high tensile strength, fungus-resistant, moth-resistant, bacteria-resistant, antistatic, heat conductive.

Texture: Soft and airy.

Therapeutic properties: Its surface texture contains breaks that create a gentle massage for the skin, stimulating circulation. Japanese researchers have reported that linen bedding used in hospitals yielded no bed sores for patients lying in hospital beds for great lengths of time. Japanese scientists concluded that better sleep and mood recovery resulted when linen bedding was used. Tests were also conducted at the Natural Fiber Institute, in Poznan, Poland. They found that through the use of linen bedding, hospital patients did not form bed sores of any kind.

Linen may reduce and help eliminate skin diseases. Medical, linen textiles were made for decubitus prevention. Wound dressings made of linen were created to heal skin ulcers. Linen keeps the ulcer at a balanced moisture level while absorbing excess exudates. Additionally, linen reduces inflammation due to the high amounts of fenolic acids and flavanoids in it. This makes the fabric antiallergenic, antiviral, and anti-inflammatory.

Sustainability: High resiliency, long life-cycle, highly renewable.

History: It was prominently produced in Russia, Asia, Belgium, and the USA. Linen was one of the first plants ever to be woven into a fabric. The silica found in flax preserves fabrics; this is why Egyptian mummies were wrapped in linen. In Egypt, it was a symbol of purity. It was also used as battle armor, called linothorax. It was also named "holy attire," and was a part of a person's sanctification path.

Availability: High availability.

LOTUS

Fabric features: Also named sacred lotus, and Chinese lotus root, it's an aquatic plant and considered a wild, invasive plant. The stems are used to make the fabric. Lotus is one of the first natural microfibers discovered. It's also a plant-based, sylk alternative. Lotus fabric is currently in minor phase production, due to the lack of technology available and the current traditional practices being used. Developing textile machinery for lotus fabric production will decrease its high cost.

Fiber characteristics: Breathable, high absorption, waterproof, quick-drying, tensile strength, stain-resistant, wrinkle-resistant, pill-resistant.

Texture: It's soft, light, silk-like, and has a glossy sheen. It feels like a linen/silk/cotton combination.

Therapeutic properties: The fabric produces a soothing, calming effect. Taken as a food and as a medicinal herb, it helps with blood circulation and supports the brain, heart, and stomach.

Sustainability: Highly renewable, fast-growing.

History: It is hand-spun using traditional Cambodian methods. The lotus is an ancient aquatic plant, popularly cultivated in water gardens. It is historically known as a spiritual symbol of purity and divine beauty. Lotus is a symbol of strength. It was traditionally used to make robes for Buddhist monks.

Availability: Moderate availability. Vast potential.

LYOCELL

Fabric features: Lyocell is a plant-based fabric made from a regenerated wood pulp from trees like eucalyptus, oak, and beechwood. Lyocell has a conversion process; some are not all healthy, but certain certifications can help with deciphering which lyocell fabrics are healthy. Its process is similar to viscose, as it uses a chemical mixture to form the pulp into a fiber, yet it's much less toxic. Tencel™ is a popular branded and patented name for lyocell.

Fiber characteristics: Breathable, hypoallergenic, moisture absorption, high tensile strength, wicking.

Texture: Soft, smooth, supple, silk-like, suede-like.

Therapeutic properties: Beechwood and eucalyptus support skin, hair, nails, and the immune system.

Sustainability: It's produced using sustainably harvested trees, and it's low-impact.

History: Lyocell was initially produced by the company American Enka in 1972. They named lyocell, Newcell. It was later produced by Courtaulds Fibers Inc., who were later named Lenzing AG in the 1980s. Lenzing named lyocell, Tencel™ in 1990.

Availability: High availability.

MILKWEED, *asclepias syriaca*

Fabric features: Milkweed is an aquatic rhizomatous plant and considered an invasive weed. The seed hair fiber is obtained from its pod. Its white filaments (also called fluff or fuzz) inside the pod can be produced as an alternative plant-down. It can be used as stuffing, padding, and for winter apparel. It can also be spun and woven into a yarn to make woven and knit fabrics. When blended with other fibers it can create a sheen.

Tests have shown that milkweed floss has the same density as goose-down, and is an even better insulator. Its hollow structure makes it similar to goose-down. The thermal impedance level of milkweed floss equals that of goose-down. The material has been tested successfully by the Canadian Coast Guard for various types of cold weather apparel.

Fiber characteristics: Hypoallergenic, moisture absorption, hydrophobicity, waterproof, low density, pest-repellent, high insulation.

Texture: Soft, cotton-like.

Therapeutic properties: It's a medicinal plant. The roots and leaves are used to support the immune system. It has a light, airy, soothing flotation effect.

Sustainability: Highly renewable, fast-growing.

History: It grows abundantly in North America and the Rocky Mountains. Native Americans used the fiber floss to line their children's cradles. Europeans wove it into fabric in the seventeenth century. It was originally used for life jackets, and as a stuffing material.

Availability: Minor availability.

NETTLE, *urtica dioica*

Fabric features: Nettle, also named European stinging nettle, is made from the fibrous stem of the plant. There

224

is also a fabric made from the Himalayan giant nettle (Giardinia diversifolia) that produces the aloo fiber. It has a hollow structure giving it natural thermal insulation and cooling properties similarly found in linen. It will soften after washing.

Fiber characteristics: Breathable, parasite-resistant, moth-repellent, wrinkle-resistant.

Texture: It has a slight glossy sheen, lustrous, and it has similar properties to linen.

Therapeutic properties: The plant is popular in herbal medicine, and is taken as an herbal supplement.

Sustainability: This fast-growing weed can be both wild-harvested and farm-harvested. Its extensive root system plays a role in the conservation of soil.

History: Most nettle textile production is in Europe. Nettle has been used for centuries in Nepal. It was very popular in medieval times. Traces of nettle fabric have been found in Denmark, and from the Bronze Age.

Availability: Minor to moderate availability.

PALMYRA PALM, *borassus*

Fabric features: Palmyra, or palm fiber, is a long staple fiber and member of the Palmae family. It's a subtropical plant. The fiber is extracted from the palm fruit.

Fiber characteristics: Moisture regain, flexibility, tensile strength.

Texture: Soft, cotton-like.

Therapeutic properties: It has anti-inflammatory properties. It supports the skin and helps eliminate infection. The fruit itself contributes to hydration.

Sustainability: A natural waste food industry by-product, highly renewable.

History: The use of the palm's oil originates in the tropics of West Africa. It's been used for thousands of years.

Availability: Vast potential.

PANDANUS, *amaryllifolius*

Fabric features: Commonly known as pandan, or screwpine, it is used mostly for accessories like bags and hats. It has vast potential to be made into an apparel fabric. An 80% cotton and 20% pandan fiber blend called Philippine Tropical Fabric (PTF) was successfully produced at the Philippine Textile Research Institute. It is commonly produced in bags, hats, mats, but also can be made into a finer thread for apparel.

Fiber characteristics: Breathable, strength, stain-resistant, low-pillage.

Texture: Soft, smooth.

Therapeutic properties: Several pandanus species are medicinal. The leaf is used as an herbal remedy. It is naturally cleansing, and a pain reliever.

Sustainability: Highly renewable, it is considered an invasive species.

History: Screwpine weaving was traditionally crafted in Kerala. It is widely used in South Asian cooking.

Availability: Moderate availability (for accessories). Vast potential (for apparel).

PINA

Fabric features: Pina fabric is made from pineapple leaves.

Fiber characteristics: Breathable, moisture-resistant, durable, strength, flexibility.

Texture: Soft, silk-like, airy, glossy, lustrous, delicate.

Therapeutic properties: Pineapple leaves are known for their medicinal value when drunk as a tea.

Sustainability: A natural waste food industry by-product.

History: Pina fabric is commonly made in the Philippines. Pina production began in the sixteenth century. It was in demand in the nineteenth century. Pina weaving is an ancient art.

Availability: Moderate availability.

PINE NEEDLE

Fabric features: The fine, inner short fibers of the pine needle can be turned into fabric, or made into a fiber composite. They contain cellulose and lignin. Its inner fibers can be made into lyocell, and also turned into a yarn/fabric. Pines needles can also be produced and used as a natural dye.

Fiber characteristics: Moisture absorption, moisture-wicking, thermoregulating, tensile strength, moth-resistant, antibacterial, antimicrobial, naturally odor-reducing, insulating.

Texture: Soft, silky, and similar to cotton.

Therapeutic properties: Taken as an herb it is anti-cancer, and it heals damaged DNA. Medicinal, natural, essential oils are within the plant material, which can be extracted and used as a textile treatment. They are naturally antibacterial and antiseptic.

Sustainability: A natural waste forest by-product, highly renewable.

History: There is current research and development of the forest by-product of pine needles and its use as a wool alternative. Pine needle viscose is already patented, but viscose is not suitable. Other products are being made from pine needles, such as blended, pine fiber composites.

Availability: Minor availability. Vast potential.

RAMIE, *boehmeria nivea*

Fabric features: Ramie, also known as China grass, is a bast/stem fiber. Ramie is named Chinese nettle, but it is different from European nettle. It's an herbaceous perennial and a member of the nettle family.

Fiber characteristics: Hypoallergenic, moisture-wicking, quick-drying, hygroscopic, absorbent, thermobalanced, high tensile strength, antibacterial, antifungal, moth-proof, stain-resistant, wrinkle-resistant.

Texture: Silky-sheen, soft, and linen-like.

Therapeutic properties: The leaves and roots can be eaten for medicinal effects and it is used for wound care.

Sustainability: Fast-growing, highly renewable.

History: It is one of the oldest crops, largely produced in China, Brazil, India, Taiwan, Korea, and the Philippines, and cultivated in subtropical areas. It was one of the top fabrics used in ancient times. Ramie was used and found covering the mummies in Egypt during 5000–3000 BC.

Availability: High availability.

ROSE

Fabric features: A cellulose bast fiber. The rose fiber is extracted from rose bushes and their stems. It takes in natural dyes easily. Rose viscose has been produced, but it needs to be produced using the lyocell textile process or other healthier fabric processes. A rose fabric made from rose petals has also been recently produced. Additionally, dyes extracted from the petals can be used to dye fabrics.

Fiber characteristics: Breathability, ventilation, moisture absorption, strength, flexibility, appearance retention, warmth.

Texture: Soft, silk-like, shiny. It's similar in appearance to a bamboo fabric's drape.

Therapeutic properties: Soothing. It contains 16 amino acids that are healthy for skin.

Sustainability: Biodegradable, a natural waste by-product.

History: Origin is not known; this is a new fabric.
Availability: Minor availability. Vast potential.

SASAWASHI
Fabric features: Sasawashi fabric is a blend of both paper and fiber. It's made from a blend of Japanese paper and fibers from the herbal Kumazasa plant. *Sasa* means "bamboo grass." *Washi* stands for paper coming from the wood pulp of trees and shrubs like kozo, mitsumata, mulberry, or gampi. Mitsumata and gampi's natural oils are used to soften the fabric's appearance, and to make it appear leathery. Most paper yarns are twisted with a fiber to give the fabric its stability.
Fiber characteristics: Thermoregulating, strength, durability, antibacterial, deodorizing, anti-allergen, anti-mildew, absorbent, anti-pillage, anti-static.
Texture: It has a soft, dry, gentle touch, and is similar to cashmere and Egyptian cotton.
Therapeutic properties: Kumazasa is a detoxifying and blood-purifying herb. It alleviates skin conditions and has anti-aging properties.
Sustainability: Highly renewable.
History: By the first half of the twentieth century, washi yarn was popularly used in Japan and Europe. Paper yarns are a lasting tradition in Japan. Its demand is increasing worldwide. Fabric woven with washi yarn is called *shifu*.
Availability: Moderate availability.

SEACELL™
Fabric features: Seacell™ is a patented textile by Smartfiber AG. It is made of lyocell with a permanently embedded seaweed powder infused into the cellulose.
Fiber characteristics: Breathable, hypoallergenic, moisture

absorption, moisture-wicking, high tensile strength.

Texture: Soft, supple, smooth, silky.

Therapeutic properties: Seacell's seaweed-infused lyocell contains minerals, trace elements, amino acids, and the vitamins A, B, and E. It is made of eucalyptus and seaweed, both of which support cell regeneration.

Sustainability: The plant is cut above the regenerative part which is used to harvest the seaweed fabric infusion treatment, to encourage the plant's growth. It has a carbon neutral production process.

History: Smartfiber AG was founded in 2005, in Germany. In addition to their patented process of embedding seaweed into cellulose, they also have a patented "Smartcel™ sensitive," cosmetic fabric made with zinc oxide. Zinc oxide supports the skin and immune system.

Availability: Moderate availability.

SILK FLOSS TREE, *ceiba/chorisia speciosa*

Fabric features: The silk floss tree contains a seed fiber, from the Malvaceae, Bombax and Baobob family. The tree contains large fruit seedpods filled with fluffy hairs similar to the fibers found in the cottonwood tree and kapok tree seedpods. The fluff can be spun into yarn and/or used as an insulator, and as a plant-down alternative.

Fiber characteristics: Buoyant, waterproof, strength, durability, thermal, insulating.

Texture: Soft, cotton-like, silk-like.

Therapeutic properties: The tree is symbolically called "the tree of refuge," and "the sheltering tree." It has a protective, as well as an airy, floating quality.

Sustainability: A natural waste by-product of the tree.

History: Native to South America, Argentina, and Brazil. Indigenous South American tribes long utilized the waterproof bark of silk floss trees to make canoes. The fiber fluff was formerly used for stuffing pillows and life jackets.

Availability: Vast potential.

SPANISH MOSS, *tillandsia usneoides*

Fabric features: Spanish moss, "tree hair," is an epiphyte. It can only grow on another plant. It is not actually a moss; it's a flowering plant. The inner part from the core is used for fabric; beneath the green covering is the fiber. Historically, this plant was used for apparel goods.

Fiber characteristics: Breathability, tensile strength, water-repellent, moisture evaporation, elasticity, anti-viral.

Texture: It's delicate and airy. It's similar to wool yet softer and lighter.

Therapeutic properties: It is taken as an herbal supplement for the heart, lung, and liver. It was also put in infants' cradles for hygienic purposes.

Sustainability: A forest by-product.

History: Native Americans like the Houma, Seminole, Alibamu, and at least 16 other indigenous groups, used Spanish moss for textile use. Insulation and padding products are currently made from Spanish moss. Saddle blankets are made from it because they do not cause skin abrasion to the horse, and it keeps the horse dry. Blankets were made out of Spanish moss by the Koasati. The Apalachee women wore skirts, tunics, and shawls made from Spanish moss.

Availability: Vast potential.

WATER HYACINTH, *eichhornia crassipes*

Fabric features: Water hyacinth is a stem fiber. The stem part of the plant is used for textile production. It is an aquatic weed available in many parts of the world. Water hyacinth was tested as a fiber blend, and was found to be successful for apparel goods, by the Department of Science and Technology's Philippine Textile Research Institute (PTRI.)

Fiber characteristics: Breathability, absorbency, tensile strength.

Texture: Soft, light and airy.

Therapeutic properties: The stem, leaf, and flower are edible. Its stem yields high amounts of potassium, and the leaves are high in protein.

Sustainability: It is an invasive species, making it a natural waste resource. It grows rapidly and abundantly in all types of freshwater. It can double its population in two weeks, making it highly renewable. Aggressive mats of water hyacinth can form in the water causing oxygen depletion. So, the harvesting of this stalk can support aquatic life. Its roots purify the water. It's an economic source for developing communities.

History: The plant is known to be native in South America.

Availability: Vast potential.

WATER LILY, *nymphaeaceae*

Fabric features: Also named Egyptian lotus, water lily fiber has important value, as it is yet another aquatic plant for textile use. The Philippine Textile Research Institute successfully developed a new textile made from water lily stems.

Fiber characteristics: Breathability, tensile strength, elasticity.

Texture: Soft, silky, glossy.

Therapeutic properties: Soothing, calming.

Sustainability: It will support economic development. It is highly renewable, and fast-growing.

History: Water lily fabric is a new fiber made in the Philippines. The water lily symbol is commonly found in ancient Egyptian tombs.

Availability: Vast potential.

WISTERIA

Fabric features: Wisteria, also named *Fujifu,* is a fabric woven and made of wisteria bark fibers. It is an ancient textile made out of wisteria vines. The fibers can be produced into a coarse to fine fabric.

Fiber characteristics: Breathable, moisture absorption, tensile strength, twice as strong as linen.

Texture: It has a silky sheen, it's soft, and is similar to hemp and linen.

Therapeutic properties: The fiber itself, and its traditional textile production process, is known for being spiritual and mystical.

Sustainability: Highly renewable, grows rapidly, an invasive weed.

History: It is found in Eastern USA, China, Korea, Japan, etc. It is one of the oldest known fabrics in Japan, dating from the prehistoric Jomon period, 14000–300 BC. Fujifu is recognized as a designated traditional handicraft in Kyoto, Niigata, and Ishikawa, Japan. It continues to be woven in a mountain village in Kyoto's Tango region.

Availability: Vast potential.

Chapter 9

Plant-based Fabric Dyes

Fabric dyes for the future

Archeologists found evidence of textiles dyed with plants and bark from the Neolithic period, around 12,000 years ago. Mineral-based pigments date back to 15000 BC. Fabric dyes were natural until 1856. The first coal tar dye was developed by William Perkin. By 1915 synthetic dyes had virtually replaced most natural dyes.

Herbal dyeing found in indigenous and contemporary cultures is traditional in practice. Plant dyes that come from herbs, plants, roots, trees, bark, flowers, seeds, leaves, fruits, vegetables, and minerals are the textile dyes of the future. Botanical dyes are made with part or all of the plant. Herbal, botanical dyes are not typically made with toxic, chemical solvents. This enables the properties of herbal dyes to perform at a medicinal level. There are so many incredible herbal dye options with specific, medicinal properties that support and help heal specific ailments.

In terms of mass-producing plant-based fabric dye, it needs to be done on a mass scale, and it's already happening to a minor degree. However, plant-derived fabric dyes are glamorized as niche-based in the media, and it is creating the misperception that it is an art/craft that cannot be carried out commercially. As an example, plant-based dye production is advertised and pictured in developing countries, showing textile workers dyeing small batches of fabric in small pots over a fire.

It's true, there is no way we can clothe 7 billion people at that rate of textile dyeing production. Additionally, there are numerous, small artisanal workshops and programs on natural textile dyeing all over the world, that are supporting natural dyeing as an art and craft. Yet these niche-based, small-batch dyeing methods don't give us the bigger picture and potential of plant-based dyes for the fashion industry at large. There is not yet enough demand for "plant-tech" dyes, but there will be.

There are companies with large-scale divisions solely dedicated to plant-based dye production, and other companies solely dedicated to exclusively producing plant-based dyes for industrial use, it is just not common. The Switzerland-based dye company, Archroma, is a clear example that plant-derived dye production for the mass market can be done. They are a large, commercial-based dye company utilizing nature's resources, creating beautiful plant-based pigments on a mass scale. They created a new, patented dye method process that produces a collection of colorants called EarthColors®. Their dyes are made from non-edible agricultural and herbal industries' natural waste, such as leaves and nutshells.

A wide range of plant-based dye colors can be made to have a bold and saturated appearance. Diluted, pale-looking dye colors do not represent the entire case of all plant-based dye colors. Natural colors and pigments on Earth are vibrant, exuberant, and can replicate synthetic dyes, depending on the textile pigment processing and plant and mineral types used. There are bright and bold dye extracts from the petals of exotic flowers, bright blues from mineral gems, bright greens from seaweed, to deep grays from mud and clay.

Sometimes, we find that some fashions do not look like high fashion when they are plant-dyed. It is not so much the fabric dye color, but the design aesthetic of a garment that majorly contributes to it being perceived as modern. Some colors of plant-based dyed fabrics appear diluted, yet there's a soothing, light, and modern feeling from them that is appealing. When the aesthetic design of a garment is successfully achieved, the garment's dye color will have a modern look, tone, and mood.

Textile dyeing methods in transition

If textile manufacturers can't produce 100% plant-based fabrics made with 100% plant-based dyes, they should produce the biodiverse, plant-based fabric varieties first and more vastly, then produce plant-based dyes second. This is in order to proceed into the fashion industry's natural, gradual progression.

Plant-based fabrics made with low-impact or plant-based dyes are more effective than polyester fabrics made with plant-based dyes. Generally speaking, if a textile manufacturer produces a synthetic textile, chances are they are not going to dye it with plant dye; they will use a petroleum/coal-based synthetic dye.

There is no appeal in dyeing polyester, nylon, and acrylic fabrics with plant-derived dyes; they just don't match or go together. For example, when essential oils are merged or heated into petroleum-based plastic, there would most likely be toxic fumes mixed with the scent of plastic emanating off the material as the plastic and essential oils are heated and rubbed together.

In order of importance, plant-based fabrics that are plant dyed will be ideal, yet plant-based fabrics dyed with low-impact dyes and semi-natural dyes are good too. Healthy, safer chemicals will be a part of the future of fashion. There is always a process for everything, and taking the necessary steps will lead to a natural product. There's a major need to develop more technology that produces plant dyes on a mass scale. There needs to be more marketing and trend value, also, towards the qualities of plant-based dyes comparable to commercially produced synthetic dyes.

Low-impact dyes

Low-impact textile dyes are highly recommended. The ultimate dye is plant-derived, yet low-impact dyes are some of the most advanced types of dyes to use, and many are certified. They are a good place to start when transitioning away from conventional dyes. Overall, low-impact dyes and semi-natural dyes are essential, but herbal, plant-based dyes are the optimal choice.

I am not going to go into great detail about low-impact dyes, yet they are seemingly the most appropriate, sufficient, and a better type of dye to use instead of generic, synthetic, petroleum-based dyes. Dyes that are low-impact are synthetic, yet involve fewer chemicals and chemical combinations that would normally be toxically potent or poisonous. So, they are gentle for human health and the environment.

Low-impact dye production eliminates heavy, toxic chemicals, reduces water usage, and causes less pollution to humans and the environment. Many sustainable and eco-friendly dyes use less water. As well, these textile dye manufacturers have methods to eliminate or reuse the used water from after-dye applications in a safe manner. If these dyes do end up in waterways, a water treatment needs to be set in place, whether the dye is healthy or non-toxic.

We can still use chemicals in our plant-based dyes, they just need to be safe and healthy. It is a matter of selecting and producing non-toxic chemicals that are helpful to the body. Several new plant-dye methods made by the textile industry will combine plants with non-toxic chemicals to make industrial textile dyes. They don't have to be 100% pure and in their natural state to be healthy. It would be quite taxing to cover all fabrics with plant dyes without having a few chemicals involved to make it possible for mass production.

Ayurvastra: dyeing fabric with medicinal, ayurvedic herbs and spices

Ayurvastra is a 5000-year-old Ancient Eastern Indian system of natural textile-dyeing. *Ayur* means "health," *vastra* means "clothing." Ayurvastra dyers dye cotton fabric with herbal plant-based dyes. Herbal fabrics promote immunity, and treat a diverse range of diseases. Studies have shown they reduce the negative symptoms of various ailments. They enhance mood and energy levels, and offer general wellness.

Herbal dyes administer healing and recovery, and they also act as a protective agent to block out harmful, environmental chemicals and pollutants. Ayurvastra is free of toxic chemicals. All natural, plant-based mordants, plant-derived dye fixatives and fabric treatments are used in the Ayurvastra textile dye manufacturing process. A few plant dyes to mention that are part of the Ayurvastra healing system: aloe, lime, henna leaves, sandalwood, neem leaves, champa flower, indigo, turmeric, haritaki, madder, pomegranate, catechu, and onion.

Indigo, for example, is a healing, Ayurvastra herbal dye known to ward off insects and bacteria. It is known to prevent and heal bleeding and injury. It has an antiseptic and astringent effect for wound cleansing and wound healing. Indigo softens fabric fibers. It also can be used to repel harsh chemicals, as studies prove it repels carbon tetrachloride. Taken as an herbal supplement, it is a potent antioxidant, antibacterial, and anticancer herb.

The traditional, healing, indigo-dyed textiles in Asia

Textile dye made from indigo tree leaves has been used medicinally since AD 660. During the Edo period, Japanese Samurai warriors dressed in a layer of indigo-dyed cotton beneath their armor and wore indigo-dyed underwear to help heal wounds and ward off bacteria. They also dyed their armor indigo. The indigo dye earned its nickname: Samurai Blue.

Dyes interact with the skin. Kendogi Nogawa, a reputable Japanese indigo dyer and fabric manufacturer, says: "In fact, it appears artisans that work with their hands dyeing with indigo all day are sick less often." Nogawa is 80 years old, in good shape, and he has testified to this statement.

Textile dyes penetrate through the skin
Fabric dyes, fabric treatments, and laundry detergents penetrate the skin, moving through layers of tissue into the bloodstream. They are then transferred throughout the body. The dyes themselves become absorbed through the skin. Fabric finishes, fabric treatments and textile dyes should be made with prevalent care and attention to help nourish the skin, without disrupting the skin's acid mantle or the body, in general.

There are many garment labels that read: "Wash separately, clothing may bleed," "Color may wash off," or "Launder with like colors." Color bleeding is a sure thing for many highly saturated fabric dye colors. Sweat will induce color bleeding of a garment. When body temperature rises, the skin's pores and sweat glands open, and the dye will then penetrate into the skin. Because of this, it is better to wear lighter colored garments if they are made with synthetic dyes and toxic chemicals.

Take a fish, for instance. The flesh of humans has similar properties to those of fish flesh. Fashion products contain chemicals similar to heavy metals that penetrate fish skin. Heavy metals are found throughout the flesh and skin of the fish. The toxic chemicals that penetrate the skin can add up and can weaken the skin and flesh of the human body.

A study revealed that essential oil, topically applied on the tip of the thumb of a person, was found in their urine 15 minutes after if it was applied. This conveys that simply wearing herbal, plant-based dyed fabric, fabric made with herbal treatments, and laundry detergents made with essential oils and plant-derived ingredients will support the body because herbal, plant-based dye alternatives give off a positive effect when they show up in the body's bloodstream.

Innovative and alternative natural dyes

Beautifully ornate, glistening colored, modern fabric dyes can be made with plant-based materials. As fashion shifts into producing more advanced "plant-tech" remedies, plant-based colorants will be more attractive, and much more modern than many of our artificial, synthetic colorants. People aren't naturally drawn to artificial colors, yet most synthetic dye hues can be found in nature. Bright, deep-colored dye extracts can be made with plants. It's instinctual to blend in with nature, but plant dyes found in nature can come in all shades and hues.

Color brings clothing to life. Modern, bright, fluorescent and neon dyes can be made plant-based and semi-plant derived. Vivid colors are important, and can be sourced and found in nature. The intrinsic and influential color palette of Earth tones is both grounding and uplifting. We needn't detract from a natural color palette of neutrals: black, white, beige, cream, and colors that are easy on the eye like navy, violet, blue, and pale light colors that lift the spirit. Generally speaking, most colors are classic, timeless, and effortless to wear.

It has been said that the textile dye process of plant-based dyeing animal-based fabrics, like wool, is easier. Many dyers claim that wool fabric takes in plant dyes very easily. The reason why is partly because when the wool fiber is produced into a textile the lanolin which is its natural barrier is stripped from wool. Plant-based fabrics have a natural moisture barrier that protects and nourishes the skin. Some claim that dyeing plant-based fabric with plant dyes can create a lack of consistency. New, non-toxic chemicals and plant-based chemicals can be developed to fix this, because plant fabrics dyed with plants naturally go together.

Types of natural, botanical, herbal fabric dyes

Below are plant dye categories with a sample palette of plant-derived dyes, and they should be made more widely available.

Not all are mentioned; there are numerous other plant-dye options available. The plant-based textile dyes listed below are either already commercially marketed with moderate to minor availability, are produced by artisans, or are produced for personal use. Almost all dyes listed have the potential to be mass produced, but several plant-derived dyes, like lichen dyes, for example, should stay niche. Plant dyes come from herbal, botanical plants, roots, bark, flowers, seeds, leaves, trees, fruits, vegetables, minerals, soil, seaweed, and more.

Tree/Plant

- pine needles
- burdock root
- grass
- acorn
- bark of phellodendron
- eucalyptus bark
- red bark
- black walnut hulls
- logwood/sappan tree
- catechu

Leaf

- mango leaf
- henna/mehndi leaf
- indigo bay leaf
- rosemary leaves
- mullein
- peach leaves
- leaves from walnut tree
- loquat leaves

Root/Rhizome
- turmeric
- rue
- madder
- sorrel
- dandelion

Flower
- lavender
- goldenrod
- rose
- hibiscus
- hyacinth

Lichens and mushrooms
Lichens have been used since ancient times in the textile dyeing craft, but they should not be sold and produced on a large scale because the forests depend on them. Hundreds of lichens have been documented for their use as textile dyes. Mushroom dyes and mushroom leathers are in development. They would have to be the edible kind to be considered healthy fashion and wearable.

Seaweed
There are over 10,000 species of seaweed. Several textile developments have been made for the production of seaweed-derived textiles and dyes.

Minerals
- copper
- silver
- gold
- crystals

Copper, silver, and gold metals are too potent to dye fabric, but they can be used sparingly, and added to dyes. For example, they will provide health benefits if they are added or made into pigments, and screen printed onto fabrics. The colored pigments from crystals can be added to screen printing inks.

Soil

Soil is rich in minerals. Depending on the soil harvest's location, the textile dye colors from soil range from earthy browns to orange reddish and blackish colors. A fashion company, Red Dirt Shirts™, have created their own soil-based textile dyeing process, and they dye their garments with dirt. The dirt is a natural, volcanic soil by-product.

Clay

Clay is a heavy type of soil. The color dyes of clay come in an array of grays, from light gray to blue-gray, and other clay colors like yellow, red, and brown. Clays are often used as a facial mask, nourishing the skin.

Food waste by-product

Most of the world's textile industry use sheep farms for their milk, meat, skin and wool. Why not utilize farms that grow and harvest food crops, and use them to make textile dyes? We can utilize the food industry's natural food waste by-products, for instance. For example, only parts of the coconut are used in the food industry, the other parts of the coconut can be used in the textile and dye industry. Additionally, millions of pounds of fruit and vegetables rot each year. Many fruits and vegetables can be turned into a powder for the textile dye manufacturing process. Imperial graduate Nicole Stjernsward has invented Kaiku, a system that turns plants into powdered paint pigments by using vaporization technology.

Fruit

- persimmon
- juniper berries
- saw palmetto berries
- citrus peel
- grapes
- pomegranate

Vegetables

- onion
- fennel
- beet
- cabbage
- carrot

Miscellaneous food

- almond shell
- cinnamon bark
- tea
- mint
- coffee

Natural plant-based mordant used in the plant-based textile dyeing process

It is essential to apply a mordant to fabric during the textile dyeing process. A mordant is a binding agent used in order to keep the dye attached to fabrics and embedded in the fibers. One option is to use plant mordants and fixatives that are entirely 100% plant-based, and naturally contain high tannins. Plant tannins are better than some heavy metal mordants which may not be as healthy and are a hazard to waterways and sea life. Yet some mineral-based mordants are healthy to use.

The powdered leaf from symplocos trees, found in the

Indonesian mountains, is a 100% plant-based mordant alternative to metal-based mordants. The tree was discovered by the botanist Georg Eberhard Rumpf. The Arbor aluminosa "aluminum tree" comes in a genus of 250 species. The traditional symplocos mordant harvesting method is to collect the tree's fallen leaves. So, it is a natural, forest waste by-product. Scientists have proven these leaves have high aluminum levels. Additionally, its dyeing process is quicker than the alum dyeing process.

In addition to symplocos, acorns and oak galls contain an excellent source of tannin. Other plant-based mordants include horse chestnuts, pine bark, walnut, roots, leaves, and fruits. Many parts of these plant mordants can also be used as fabric colorants. Acorns, oak galls, and pomegranate rinds increase color saturations and brighten natural dyes while improving their colorfastness. Also, new "plant-tech" technology can utilize these plant mordants, and add additional plant-based ingredients to them for textile dye development.

Natural mordants for herbal healing

- myrobalans
- rhubarb leaves
- oils
- minerals
- alum
- bark of lodhra
- kenduka
- fruit extracts of haritaki
- terminalia chebula

A few more natural mordants that can also be used as a fabric treatment for health

- juniper leaves
- sumac leaves

- mango bark extract
- myrobalan
- rhubarb leaves
- castor oil
- vinegar
- avocado pits
- sumac trees
- eucalyptus barks
- juniper needles

Fabric treatments/infusions

Fabric treatments can create a fabric with specific healing textile properties. These fabric treatments/infusions create a cosmetic fabric, also known as cosmetotextiles. There are a plentiful number of options for textile treatments to support the fabric's performance along with treating the body topically, for hygiene, health, and wellbeing. A few are listed below:

Zinc is an essential trace element that supports detoxification and human skin rejuvenation. It reduces odors, resists skin infection, and is antibacterial. Fabric with zinc-infused finishing treatments may also help eliminate skin disorders like eczema.

Sea salt can help set dye in fabrics. Sea salts are tiny "crystals." Crystals are known to enhance and amplify positive energy. Sea salt is known for its healing, purification, and protective properties. It contains over 21 trace minerals essential for the body.

Castor oil is an exceptional treatment to soften skin and fabrics. This plant-based oil will help support the skin, and it has antimicrobial effects. Additionally, the fatty acids of the oil help to prevent the fabric from creasing and wrinkling.

Other textile treatments for cosmetic fabrics

- **Mint-infused fabric** used as a fabric treatment has antibacterial, cooling properties.
- **Pearl-infused fabric** is a pearl powder infused into cellulose fibers. Pearls contain eight essential amino acids and trace elements.
- **Neem oil fabric treatment** is a gentle, antimicrobial agent.
- **Linseed oil fabric treatment** is an antimicrobial agent.
- **Copper-infused fabric** supports injury and arthritis. It's known to protect the energy body.

PART 4

THE PLANT-BASED FASHION GUIDE: A HEALTHY WARDROBE AND A HEALTHY FASHION INDUSTRY

Chapter 10

What to Wear in Transition: The Transition from Conventional Fashion, to Sustainable Fashion, to Healthy Fashion

What fabrics to wear in transition

Synthetic fabrics

There's an inevitable need for consumers to purchase synthetic fabric options because that's what is currently available on the market, and because 100% cotton fashions are decreasing in many fashion retailers. Cotton is great; it's never going away. It may also be, for the most part, the bulk of many plant-based wardrobes for a while.

The high demand for synthetic fabric and the lack of plant-based apparel for all seasons make it challenging to have a wardrobe free of synthetic fabrics. But given the time, energy, and resources, it can be done. A plant-based wardrobe will become more achievable when more brands offer a variation of different plant-based fabrics, and gradually increase plant-based apparel options and the accessibility to purchase them.

A minimal amount of synthetic apparel should be worn. If the fashions are synthetic, they need to be designed ergonomically, and not create discomfort. The cut of the synthetic-based garment should be ergonomic, and the silhouette should be loose on the body. Sometimes, it is healthier to wear an ergonomic fashion design made with synthetic fabric, rather than a non-ergonomic fashion design that is made with plant-based fabrics.

Synthetic garments should be made with the most ergonomic synthetic fabrics that don't create clamminess, or itch the skin. Comfort is crucial. We need to choose ergonomic textures, and fabrics with an ergonomic feel of the fabric. The texture of the synthetic fabric should be tactile-friendly and comfortable. Many synthetic fabrics make the skin feel clammy and sweaty when the fabric and skin is rubbed together. This is not a therapeutic feeling. Whenever possible, undergarments and first-layer pieces that directly touch the skin should be plant-based. Additionally, garments with a blended fiber content—like a poly/cotton blended fabric—is better than wearing 100% synthetic fabric.

If it's not organic fabric, it doesn't mean it's unhealthy

Cotton, linen, hemp, and lyocell are some of the most prominent, leading natural fabrics currently on the market, and they don't need to be 100% organic in order to be healthy. Many farmers harvesting plant crops for textiles use chemical fertilizers and pesticides, but only use a little, and that is OK. It's easy to say "Don't wear toxic apparel, choose organic apparel." But it's not practical for most of the population today to wear 100% organic apparel. Converting entirely to an organic, plant-based wardrobe would be ideal but it is not critical. The obstacles that prevent people from converting to all-organic plant-based apparel are price, location, sourcing, and a lack of all-season plant-based apparel options.

Additionally, being ready to change psychologically plays a large role. We are so used to synthetic garments, it has been a part of our survival for so long. If a synthetic garment is really special, inspiring, and comfortable, we will still wear it or buy it, especially if they are blended with natural fibers. When we make or have a connection with synthetic, or semi-synthetic apparel, it makes it hard for us to not buy it or wear it.

Wearing Bt cotton is better than wearing 100% polyester, nylon and acrylic

Bt cotton, rather than synthetic materials, should be worn for now, at least if that is what is most accessible or available. Whenever possible, genetically modified textiles shouldn't be supported, and it only creates a vicious cycle of producing more of it when it continues to be purchased. Based on what is most important, it's plant materials over synthetic, petroleum-based materials. This does not include plant fibers that are sugar-derived, like genetically modified Ingeo™ (corn) fabric, which comes from a plant but the corn is broken down producing an acidic-promoting fabric.

At this point, there's not really an option to rule out Bt cotton 100% because of the genetically modified cotton seeds that have taken over the cotton farm industry. It was created because the Bt cotton seed produces its own insecticide, designed to combat the bollworm. It's not completely healthy due to plant seed alteration and the use of synthetic, toxic chemical-based weed, fungus and pest killer sprays farmers use on the crops to enable them to grow. It's very challenging to get away from Bt cotton at this point, yet there are options.

Consumers are bombarded with genetically modified fabric. They have infiltrated into life with very little mention of them being genetically modified. Improper labeling causes this lack of awareness. Stating "GMO-free" on a garment's content label will decrease the demand and production of Bt cotton. This may be in effect in the future, since the food industry currently labels and regulates many food products as "GMO-free" or "Non-GMO" for clarification and awareness.

Labeling "GMO" or "Non-GMO" on fabric tags or labels will alert more caution of the potential consequences and unethical plant manipulation of cotton. At this point, there is no guarantee that consumers will be able to trace the source and content of their fabrics. But if a fiber is genetically modified, it should be spelled out clearly; it's not the consumer's responsibility to detect it.

The ever-growing demand for genetically modified crops keeps them placed in the market. There isn't a fast way around this until businesses create a demand for non-GMO, natural, plant-based fabrics. Consumers can use their purchase power to enable the demand for healthier fashion.

The plant-based fashion guide: healthy wardrobe alternatives

We are at a time where we are surrounded by shopping malls. Big, corporate companies make it easy to grab-and-go. The growth of online shopping will support our need for a healthy wardrobe. There may be a few select retailers within an area or nearby city that carry healthy fashion, but there are thousands of online shops carrying healthy apparel and accessories. A quick search online and a needed product is only a click away.

E-retailers can introduce temporary pop-up shops monthly, quarterly, or yearly, in their surrounding locations, to give people another way to purchase their product, and to entice them. Their clients will have more trust and loyalty when they can try their product on, touch the fabrics, and get to know their cuts, styles, seasonal collections, and see the product face on.

For those who don't like to shop online, there are many big retailers that carry healthy fashion. It isn't always necessary to try to purchase fashion from small-end shops and specialty stores that carry only a limited selection of healthy fashion. Our needs can be met by commercial shops. Their prices are reasonable and the product is appealing. It's a matter of looking at product labels and searching for the correct fits, and so on.

Healthy alternative fabrics

Plant-tech fabrics are far more highly effective than current, popular synthetic fabrics like polyester, nylon, acrylic, and rayon.

Several alternative, plant-based fabrics to look out for:

- cotton
- linen
- hemp
- natural bamboo
- ramie
- nettle
- kapok
- kenaf
- pina
- banana
- lyocell
- jute
- sisal
- seacell™
- cork
- paper
- coconut

All of these fabrics can be produced in light, medium, and heavy fabric weights. They can be woven, braided or knitted. They can be made into different fabric types like jersey, lace, organza, sateen, satin, fleece, velvet, terry, ripstop, terry cloth, and so on. Furthermore, they can be made to withstand all-weather temperatures for maximum performance, depending on how they're made. It's a matter of more textile technology development.

Ultimately, to feed the body on the outside the way the

body is fed on the inside, it is best to wear a variety of plants. Multiple types of plants made into fabrics are essential for the environment, health, economy, social balance, and much more. Wearing only one plant, presumably cotton, won't lead to global balance.

Plant-based fabrics for cold weather

There is a plethora of warm, outdoor apparel options made of synthetic and wool fabric available, and a lack of plant-based thermal apparel. However, there are several thermal plant-based fabrics that outperform synthetic-based and animal-based thermal fabrics. These plant fabric varieties are not yet widely available on the market, but they have great potential for future and current textile developments.

Of course, it is better to stay warm in polyester and wool coats if plant-based thermal fabrics are not available. It doesn't matter what fabrics we wear that provide the necessary warmth; the body needs to stay mildly warm at all times. Thermo-regulating and thermobalanced fabrics are needed to help keep the body at a balanced temperature of primarily 37 degrees Celsius. It is better to be warm than cold. Warm clothing is a form of heat therapy, keeping the body's bones, muscles, and tendons less stiff, and the blood circulatory system functioning.

All of our internal organs and the internal structure of the body are warm, never cold, so we need to protect and stabilize our internal warmth. A dead corpse is cold to the touch. Being exposed to cold temperatures at length has health-damaging effects. Cold temperatures restrict blood flow, strain the heart, and affect blood circulation. It is uncomfortable to be cold and it disrupts the mood immediately.

Thermoregulation balance needs to be constant within cold-weather apparel. About 90% of heat is lost through the skin. The body has a way of losing and producing heat throughout the day. When it's cold we don't want to lose heat. That is why much of synthetic-based apparel is popular; they are very unbreathable, thus trapping in heat. Many thermal-based synthetic fabrics do not have moisture transport properties, thus creating trapped moisture when an individual actively sweats. Synthetic garments, when worn loose enough, can hold in heat, but still allow the body to breathe.

Plant-based thermal options for a complete, plant-based wardrobe

Plant-based options for cold weather:

- cotton and bamboo fleece
- kapok filling in puffed or quilted apparel items
- cotton or linen flannel fabric
- organic cotton batting
- waxed cotton puff jackets made with cotton batting or bamboo filling
- lining coats with organic cotton or bamboo fleece
- a plant-based faux-fur lined coat
- parkas and coats lined with milkweed or kapok plant down
- double-faced sweatshirt or terry fabric
- new, fabric layer technology
- using milkweed, cattail, flower-down, or kapok, and turning them into a thinsulate or primaloft-style fabric
- cotton chenille yarn is a soft, velvety yarn for knitwear, sweaters, heavy socks, and so on
- knitwear made with paper yarn
- biosynthetic fabric with a protective coating could be used for some outdoor apparel, and mock our favored synthetic apparel items like raincoats, and the outer shell of winter jackets and coats

Plant-down: There is a tremendous opportunity for plants such as kapok, cattails, milkweed, and silk floss tree to triumph over poly-fills and goose-down. Kapok fiber fill, for example, is an optimal alternative to feather-fill and poly-fill. Kapok fill yields extreme thermal properties. It is warmer than wool and six times lighter. Plant-down fill provides exceptional thermoregulation for indoor and outdoor apparel. If plant-down isn't available, poly-fill cannot compete with feather-fill and down-fill, in terms of their warmth.

Wind resistant/windproof textiles: Coir and cork fabrics with naturally waxed finishes have wind-resistant and water-resistant properties. They are a great alternative to synthetic fabric treatments. Biobased or biosynthetic plant-based fabrics are also wind resistant and windproof.

Waterproof textiles: Cotton ripstop with a natural wax finish and biobased synthetics with natural wax treatments are examples of plant-based waterproof textiles. Beeswax and coconut wax can be used as waterproof textile finishes. For industrial use, researchers have developed a waterproof finish made of carnauba wax, also called Brazil or palm wax, which is made from the leaves of the carnauba palm. More natural wax finish varieties need to be made.

Nylons: Plant-sylk nylons, biobased nylons, and tights/leggings made of cotton or other plant-based fabrics.

Plant "sylk": Aloe vera, rose petal, and banana can be made into a sylk fabric.

Stretch fabrics: Biobased lycra (spandex), instead of petroleum-based lycra, should be incorporated in all stretch-based fabrics. However, leggings made of 95% cotton and 5%

petroleum-based lycra leggings are much healthier and more comfortable, compared to 100% polyester leggings.

Swimwear and surf apparel: Swimwear is primarily synthetic-based. Cotton and hemp made of cotton jersey knit with biobased lycra material is preferred, or biobased synthetic swimwear. Plant-based rubber/neoprene wetsuits are an alternative to petroleum-based neoprene wetsuits. Petroleum-based neoprene is non-biodegradable. It was originally used to line the bottom of landfills, which illustrates why it may not be healthy to wear. Yulex is a neoprene, made of natural rubber from trees. A yulex wetsuit is currently available.

Eco footwear: There's an assortment of footwear fabrics and materials like lyocell, yucca, raffia palm leaves, plant-based faux leather, cork, linen canvas, and cotton canvas. These are just a few great alternatives to petroleum-based or leather footwear.

Glitter alternative: Mica sand, an organic mineral, is a glitter alternative. It has a soft, glistening, reflective, glittery appearance. It's a mineral which can be used to replace synthetic glitter. Mica can be found in beauty products for skin improvement, can be added to textile pigments to screen print on fabrics, or used as a fabric finish for apparel and accessory items.

Healthy jewelry: Costume jewelry is mostly made of plastic and artificial materials. Jewelry should consist of precious metals, gems, minerals, and soft, flexible fabric. More fabric jewelry should be included as it's ergonomic and comfortable to wear.

Non-ergonomic jewelry can disrupt the body, irritate the skin, or make the body sweat or become chilled. In the case of precious metals like copper, gold, and silver, and crystals, when they are designed correctly for the body they do enhance mood and energy levels.

Ergonomic jewelry can be made from the following materials:

- metal
- hemp
- wood
- pearl
- sisal
- jute
- plant-based leathers
- carved bamboo
- coconut shell
- crystals/gems
- seashell
- cotton weave/braided
- crocheted materials
- recycled paper
- natural tree resins

Ancient fashion meets modern fashion: inspirational, plant-based fashions from ancient cultures around the world

Many ancient cultures around the world have naturally infused healing powers in their dress for inner and outer balance, as well as for mental, physical, emotional and spiritual health.

For the purpose of uprooting the ancient healing powers found in ancient clothing for modern use, below is a small descriptive palette of fashions from countries and cultures. Several of these fashions are still being used today, and should be made prominent within the whole world, for their modern, healing, "plant-tech" significance. They made practical use of materials made primarily from plants and minerals. Additionally, we can incorporate and use these ancient fashions as part of universal fashion.

Egypt

Egyptians wore linen and ramie predominantly. Egyptians had healthy flax crop harvests along the Nile river. Flax was one of the most breathable fabrics available to them and supported their body in the warm climate. They believed animal-based fabrics were impure to wear. If they were worn, they were forbidden in sanctuaries and temples.

Egyptian rulers found as mummies in tombs from 5000 BC were wrapped in linen. When Tutankhamen's tomb was opened, ancient linen curtains were still intact. This goes to show how well linen preserves. Egyptian mummies can be seen wrapped in ramie fabric for spiritual purposes.

They made plenty of use of accessories for body adornment. Neck collars, armlets, wristlets, anklets, and headdresses were made of gems, precious metals and other natural materials. They were used to attract the "gods" to them, and for divination communication. Egyptians were fascinated by gold jewelry. Gold symbolized the sun and their connection to God. It was used as a healing modality, and represented immortality seemingly because it doesn't oxidize or corrode over time. They also used specific gems in their accessories like carnelian, turquoise, emerald, pearl, and lapis lazuli. They were designed into intricate patterns inspired by nature.

Egyptians enhanced their beauty and created art with their makeup. They used minerals and clays to produce makeup like crushed malachite and ochre for lipstick, henna for lips and eyes, black kohl for eyeliner, and blue and green eyeshadow made from minerals crushed into powders.

Major historical Egyptian hieroglyphics revealed the cat-eye technique and makeup that were applied on the Egyptians' faces and other parts of their body. The Egyptian cat-eye look was popularly used. Many of Ancient Egypt's deities such as Mafdet, Basdet, and Sekhmet were cat inspired. Additionally, black eye paint was used to protect their eyes from the sun, to ward off infection, and used as a direct defense from the "evil eye."

Israel

During biblical times, Israelites used Mediterranean plants with advanced dyeing techniques. Three-thousand-year-old textiles dyed with indigo and madder root from Israel were discovered.

The early Hebrew temple clothing from Israel was made to be a reflection of the holiness of their temples. They designed fashions that mirrored and were influenced by the design and architecture of their holy temples. The Ancient Israelites designed clothing to cover and shelter the body in order to keep their "light" in their body, and to protect the body from losing its light. They shredded and burned their clothing with the temple's menorah. It was a sacred ritual they performed when clothing became dirty to the point where it was soiled.

Mexico

Yucca, palm, and maguey were a few of the Mexicans' staple plant-based fabrics. They used minerals such as gold and silver thread. Fabric materials native to Mexico were ixtle, lechuguilla, reeds, palm, twigs, and willow. Zigzags, spirals, stepped frets, moon phase shapes, plants, animals, crosses, flowers and geometry were common fashion motifs used in their embroidery and loom woven fabrics.

Guatemala

The traditional dress in Guatemala is called traje, and it

originated from their Mayan ancestors. Bold shades of color and highly energizing fabric prints were produced. Esoteric design symbols were woven into fabrics that executed the Mayan vision. Their fabrics had sacred meanings that were expressed through color, symbol, pattern, and geometric designs.

They typically used the backstrap loom to create woven patterned textiles. Guatemalan weavers would weave their own nahual sign, their animal spirit, into the fabric. The nahual is also named: Mayan sign, Mayan spirit, and nawal. Nahual signs are based from the Mayan horoscope, the symbols were used to watch over and protect them, and it was to give spiritual guidance to a person's path.

A myth of the Mayans: Grandmother of the Moon, the goddess Ixchel, taught the first woman how to weave at the beginning of time. For 3000 years many Guatemalan mothers have taught their daughters how to weave.

Aztec and Mayan

The Aztecs are known for their weaving. Colorful, loom woven fabrics were made as an art form. The Goddess Ix Azal Uoh was called the "weaver of life," and was known as a symbol of the sacred spirit within all. They favored bark-cloth and hemp fabrics. Natural indigo dye was prominently used and it was considered sacred. Brocade cloth belts and embroidered belts were a spiritual embellishment for their garments. They intertwined pieces of cloth within their hair and used headdress turbans. Fringe and knots were popular elements in their fashion. They used sea shells, metallic discs, seeds, pods, petals, crystals of jade, amber, quartz, and other natural materials in their designs to symbolize and evoke nature, spirit and health.

Parashuram and the Sages

"Valkal" fabric was made by beating the leaves and bark of the banyan tree, or pipal fig tree. Parashuram and the Sages wore flowers, lotus, leaves, and seeds. They wore lots of jewels and cotton with gold threads interwoven in fabrics. Gold metal embedded and woven into threads is still being done today, and is used in embroidery.

Native Americans

Native Americans produced apparel based on the different climates and regions they inhabited like the tropical regions, desert regions, woodland mountains, and the arctic tundra. They lived in harmony with nature, and it was reflected in their fashion.

Historically, the weaving instrument was first developed in AD 1200, by the Native Americans.

Tree bark was one of their main natural sources that they used to make fabric. It was stripped, dried, and shredded. Due to it being abundantly renewable, they could easily discard and make new bark cloth. A few types of bark cloth textiles came from cedar, sagebrush, mulberry and redwood trees, and bushes. They produced twine from milkweed, and used it to bind and sew hides, clothing and footwear. Cotton and agave were a couple of their top choice plant-based fabrics. Fringe, beadwork, and embroidery were incorporated in their fashions.

Apparel and accessory healing modalities in fashion as specific forms of therapy

Here are a few examples of progressive apparel and accessory healing modalities that are for therapeutic and medicinal use:

Healing/protective jewelry: Copper, metal, magnets.

Fashion for air flow: Gauze, breathable mesh, knitted belts.

Natural heat-producing scarf: The "heat wrap" is a knit-based heating wrap I designed. It is made without electricity or any device. You can wear it as an accessory, and also use it like it's a heating pad. It naturally heats up the body quickly. It is a 13-foot knit scarf. Due to its length, once wrapped around certain parts of the body it brings instant heat to the affected area. Because it is made with a slightly loose knit, the wrapped layers have many air sockets, which is an additional ergonomic property of the heat-producing scarf.

Weighted fabrics: Weighted shawl wraps, and other garments filled with a weighted natural substance, can be worn daily to alleviate certain conditions like stress and anxiety. They are often used medically, as a treatment for the autistic. The weight of the product pulls the body down, which reduces muscle tension and soothes the nervous system. Weighted fabrics and fashion designs can also strengthen weakened muscles, and can be used as a form of physical therapy.

Flotation-influenced fashions: Flotation fabrics defy gravity. They increase cellular communication within the body, and can even support higher states of consciousness. They produce a purifying, freeing, weightless effect. Puff jackets, even made with poly-fill, for example, can produce a levitation effect. All gravity-defying fashions can be used as a form of physical therapy. They relax the mind and body, making people feel more positive.

Acupressure apparel: Acupressure apparel worn daily can definitely help relieve pain, and also support chronic health conditions. Acupressure points work with the body's meridian channels. The meridians channel the flow of energy. They support the brain, organs, and the entire body. Acupressure apparel like shoes with acupressure points, gloves made with acupressure points, and more acupressure clothing like acupressure hats, clothing, and accessories need to be developed more.

Orgonite jewelry

Orgonite was developed in 1940 by Wilhelm Reich. Orgonite contains a mix of crystals, metals, and resin compressed in a mold. This blend creates a piezoelectric effect, making it electrically polarized. It is used to unblock and transmute negative energy in the body and environment. It is said to amplify universal life-force energy. Orgonite is a healing tool to combat negative energy. Orgonite transmutes harmful, carcinogenic radiation and electrical smog from electronic devices. The body is in a perpetual state of stress from electrical radiation alone. It strengthens the immune system, and is a pathogen-resistant compound. Additionally, orgonite emits purifying, negative ions into the air.

A study was carried out by about 30 professors; they researched the effects of orgone on cancer. Over the course of 4 years there was a 75% reduction in cancer cell growth using orgone as a natural anticancer treatment. For beneficial effects, orgonite can be used in fabrics and fashion accessories.

Monoatomic gold/ormus

Ormus gold incorporated into fabrics, textile dyes, and fashion accessories like shoes, bags, hats, and jewelry provides health-fortifying effects. Ancient Egyptians, Sumerians, Israelites, Minoans, Peruvians, Incans, Eastern Indians, and Etruscans used ormus, also named monoatomic gold, for its health-promoting and spiritually benefiting properties. Ormus supports health, healing, aging, mood, and energy levels. Ormus gold is also used to heal wounds and infection when placed on the body.

In different cultures, gold was/is a symbol of the sun, and

they even worshipped it. The sun also symbolizes the heart of each human. The "Great Central Sun" is the source and the center of the all-pervading presence of the great "I Am." The sun is a vortex, a point of integration, and also called the origin of science and the spirit of creation. Like the frequency of the sun, the ormus' frequency is a point of balance between negative and positive frequencies.

Monoatomic gold (ormus) consists of "transition" elements that are a state between pure matter and energy. Experiments show that ormus levitates, making it a supernatural mineral. As it defies gravity it makes the body feel lighter at the atomic level. Like crystals, ormus and gold are energy conductors, removing heavy, residual energies.

Food-grade ormus in the form of a powder or liquid is taken internally for healing and rejuvenating benefits. Studies have proved that 38 out of 40 people with cancer that were treated with Ormus M3 fully recovered. High concentrations of ormus are found in aloe vera, carrots, gingko, bloodroot, blue-green algae, and concord grapes, all of which can be used as textile dyes.

Healing plant- and mineral-based beauty and hygiene products

There's no healthy fashion without healthy hair, makeup, and hygiene. The fashion and beauty industry go hand in hand. As they merge, an ultimate healing fashion ensemble occurs. Without a comfortable-feeling appearance, there's a lack of health. There's a large number of toxic products being used in the fashion and beauty industry. To achieve overall health, natural non-toxic products are an important part of fashion, making one feel fresh and modern.

This quick list below contains alternative, natural hygiene and beauty products for males and females. They create a holistic, healthy fashion picture. It includes the most beautifying, revitalizing, and powerful healing remedies for daily maintenance of body, mind, and soul. They will make you feel and look great.

All-natural health retailers and natural food stores carry plant and mineral-based products. Listed below are a few of the basic ingredients of beauty and hygiene products, that are the ultimate for mind/body/spirit:

Skin

- natural exfoliation brushes andok fix prev scrubs using plant-based materials that are plastic-free
- skin moisture mists: flower water spray mist, essential oil mixed with water and/or oil
- body wash: Dead Sea salt, clay blends, glycerin and castor oil-based products
- plant oils for skin: almond, rose, rosehip, apricot, jojoba, olive, and palm oil
- antifungal: tea tree, peppermint, geranium and eucalyptus essential oils

Facial

- witch hazel
- rose water
- honey masks
- bentonite clay
- gem elixirs
- flower essence

Spa bath products

- sea salt
- Epsom salt
- hydrogen peroxide
- baking soda
- borax

Non-toxic lip care

- coconut oil
- cocoa butter
- beeswax
- primrose oil
- vitamin E oil
- balms cured with herbs

Hair

- hair conditioning: amla oil, aloe vera hair mask
- natural hair dyes: semi-permanent with naturally-derived ingredients, or low-impact boxed dyes

Teeth

- fluoride-free toothpaste
- essential oils
- aloe vera
- turmeric/black pepper mouthwash
- sesame oil gargle

Cosmetics/Makeup

- mineral-based
- botanical-based
- clay-based

Natural fragrance

- aromatherapeutic essential oils
- Ancient Roman perfumes were made of saffron, rose petals, lilies, myrtle, laurel, and jasmine.
- Holy anointing oil is a spiritual fragrance that creates an aura of holiness. It's from Israel and is made of olive oil and spices such as myrrh, cinnamon, calamus, and cassia.

Natural clothing care

Clothing care is an important part of fashion. Laundry detergents play a critical role for health and wellbeing. Without natural laundry treatments, clothes are not healthy. They are a necessary component of personal hygiene. Toxic chemicals found in detergents, fabric softeners, and fabric brighteners pollute the body. The skin absorbs the harsh, toxic-laden synthetic detergents made with unnatural substances. They cause rashes, microbial issues, infection, and autoimmune disorders.

Plant-derived detergents clean the garments but also directly support, protect and nourish the skin. There has recently been a rise in hypoallergenic laundry detergents that are safer for the skin and environment. Hypoallergenic, synthetic-free, and synthetic fragrance-free detergents include plant-based and non-toxic mineral-based ingredients. Some include all-natural fragrance made purely from essential oils.

Toxic synthetic detergents

In 1916, the first synthetic detergent was made in Germany. Chemical scientists created petrochemicals due to a shortage of the fat and oil that was primarily used to make laundry soap. Petrochemicals are synthetic chemicals found in petroleum and are added to thousands of products and materials to date. Petroleum-based products were produced for the mass market starting in the early to mid 1930s. The American company Procter and Gamble introduced its first synthetic detergent in 1930. Before this, regular soap was used as a detergent.

Monsanto, recently acquired by Bayer, was the top leading and founding chemical manufacturer of genetically modified products and chemicals. A major synthetic detergent brand, "All," was made by Monsanto in the 1940s. "All" detergent and other leading detergents like Tide, Downey, Gain, and so on, are made with harsh chemicals, dyes, fragrances, and such like. These detergents can harshly irritate the body and weaken the immune system.

Case studies show that several diseases and ailments are caused by synthetic detergents. The diseases and ailments caused by synthetic detergents include: endocrine disruption, pneumonia, cancer, neurological disorders, skin rashes, asthma attacks, allergies, respiratory failure, immunity malfunction, hormone disruption, kidney and liver disease, brain toxicity, fetal development disruption, and more. Additionally, the chemicals are inhaled into the lungs and respiratory system, affecting the nervous system by day and night.

According to the EPA, one third of scented detergents contain at least one chemical that can potentially cause cancer. Many harsh chemicals are found in synthetic laundry detergent, like sodium lauryl sulfate, ammonia, echo glare, phenols, phosphates, phthalates, sodium hypochlorite, nonylphenol ethoxylates, and quaternium-15. They are all carcinogenic toxins, and none of them are required to be listed on the product label.

Synthetic detergents and dryer sheets have a leaching property and an ability to encase a semi-permanent to permanent chemical residue on fabrics. Additionally, they can create a film on them. This film readily absorbs into the skin and bloodstream. Look at skin moisturizers that rapidly disappear and absorb in the skin within seconds after topical application. This is what the detergents on a garment's fabric can do, when the fabric rubs against the skin.

Synthetic detergents that leave a residue on fabric can be compared to the cigarette smoke that permanently embeds in car upholstery, carpet and hard surfaces. Humans are no longer wearing just fabrics, they are wearing detergent. Additionally, instead of "secondhand smoke," it's "secondhand detergent."

There is no easy way to evacuate the detergent smell. The detergent can embed, absorb, merge and blend into a fiber composition permanently or semi-permanently. This is invasive to the fabric and also to the body. Natural laundering treatments absorb into the skin, and are beneficial, without causing any harm or toxic scent.

It can take minutes, days, months, or years to see or feel the negative results of using toxic products. This is due partly to the levels of human desensitization and human conditioning. It's also caused by the rampant amount of chemicals that humans are exposed to daily. Health issues and chronic allergies caused by synthetic detergent may go unnoticed. If a person's health is declining or they have a depleted immune system, toxic detergents may leave people irritated, aggravated, and it may worsen the condition.

Healthy laundering products

Healthy detergent ingredients include plant-based surfactants and plant-based enzymes that clean the fabrics. Detergents made with essential oils, herbal extracts, and natural fragrance are a healthy substitute for artificial fragrance. Soapwort is a natural laundry detergent and good to use for textile preservation. Detergent made with sea salt is another effective laundry product to nourish the skin. Sea salt hydrates and mineralizes skin, with several other benefits.

A bleach alternative is hydrogen peroxide. It's a natural stain remover and brightener that whitens whites, and is much safer and gentler than chlorine bleach. It can be used to spot-clean stains, remove odors, and it cleans and disinfects. Additionally, baking soda and water can be used as a fabric cleanser and natural fabric brightener.

Borax, a brand name for "boron," is the salt of boric acid, and is a mineral. It is a chosen product for household cleaning and as a laundry booster. It can whiten, brighten, and cleanse fabric, and naturally soften the fabric and skin. Additionally, its mineral content can help humans, as the body is typically mineral deficient, so Borax used topically could be a potential form of mineral supplementation.

Borax is gentle to skin and fabric, not abrasive. It has a natural, slightly acidic pH level. The skin needs to be slightly acidic to keep unwanted bacteria away. Borax is commonly used for wound management. If it helps to heal a wound when taken internally or externally, it can also enhance, protect, and recover skin conditions when administered through laundering.

Natural clothing care essentials

Chalk removes oil stains. A stain remover made of mixed clays is 100% natural with no solvents. It removes grease stains, which are some of the most challenging fabric stains to get rid of. Oil and grease stains on clothing are a huge waste factor, as stains make a garment unwearable.

A garment steamer is a great way to remove wrinkles if there's no time to iron clothing. Not only does it take just seconds to heat up, the steamer is an effortless way to remove wrinkles from clothing. Unless clothing is in bad shape and needs to be ironed, most garments need a quick steam taking only minutes, and they come out flawless. This can also be a way to freshen up clothing that has already been worn, but isn't dirty.

For garment preservation, garment bags made with natural cotton and linen are an option. When clothes are unworn for a season or several seasons and preserved in bags, they have a longer life cycle. Additionally, repurposing, mending, and upcycling will instill a deeper sense of the fashion/human connection between style, fashion, and self.

Supporting green, eco-friendly laundromats and dry cleaners is an alternative to generic laundromats that pollute. Laundromat dryer vents pollute the Earth, releasing over 25 volatile compounds hazardous to the environment and humans.

People have reported lung issues caused by laundromats. Lungs can become tight, unable to take in air naturally from exposure to synthetic detergents. Additionally, one single wash of a synthetic garment yields 700,000 microscopic plastic fibers into the environment, a study finds. Another factor, studies have estimated that there are 92 to 236 metric tons of microplastics found in the ocean. They are released into waterways by laundry drains.

A feng shui wardrobe

The top shops for a feng shui wardrobe are eco, sustainable, organic, resale, vintage, recycled, designer, e-shops, retail apps, boutiques, green shops, high fashion retailers, or luxury designers. Secondhand shops are a green alternative in order to reduce waste. What makes shopping and finding clothes more precious and sentimental is when clothing is hunted for, it becomes a treasure.

Being selective will naturally come about through the practice of healthy fashion wardrobe shopping. Taking time to be aware of products positively affects how we look. Self-awareness through wardrobe shopping creates beauty. The creativity of shopping improvisation provides more intuitive fashion selections. Wardrobe curation is healthy, and will make individual style much more cultivated, rather than garment collecting. Making purposeful, conscious decisions is stylish.

It's never easy to rummage through dresser drawers to find an outfit. Lots of clothing waste accumulates when clothing is tucked away in drawers or closets. Things can eventually get piled together. If it's out of sight it's out of mind. This may lead to buying more clothing because of closets and drawers that have a lack of visual exposure. Clear bins or exposed shelving are effective. Clothing can be incorporated into a room; exposed wardrobes are current. Keeping a decorative dressing rack with shelving helps with mindfulness and organization.

It also saves time.

It's difficult to select clothes from the wardrobe when things start to pile up. There's also a feeling of waste when clothing hasn't been worn enough, or if it was an impulse purchase, and the garments don't get worn. Recycling is a reasonable excuse to remove excess clothing and it serves as a huge conductor for healthy living.

Getting rid of clothing is easier said than done. The fewer things that are hung on to, the more efficient and easy life becomes. Any clothing that hasn't been worn in over a month, excluding seasonal items or special occasion looks, should be sent to a thrift store. Selling on consignment or donating works as well.

Getting rid of an item is sometimes challenging, yet also freeing. It makes kept clothing more precious and attention-worthy. It makes select pieces truly wanted to be worn and expressed. Getting rid of clothing helps to declutter the mind. One can become either a collector or a hoarder. Collecting clothes isn't bad if it's a hobby. Creating a feng shui, minimal wardrobe is an optimal choice if you are not a collector. Minimalism is a part of eco living. Less clothing can equal more efficiency.

Healthy fashion wardrobe and style essentials

The power of clothing essentially lies behind the intention of a person's fashion. Self-awareness through personal dress creates beauty and inspiration. When we take the time to be aware of selecting garments through improvisational, mindful shopping, this positively affects how we look, and a person's style will be much more cultivated. Making purposeful, conscious decisions affects the mind and body positively. Rather than collecting a large, chaotic, collection of clothes, a small, careful curation of clothing is better. The pursuit of rash purchases provides meaninglessness and emptiness. Having a close relationship with clothing sometimes means having fewer clothes. It makes the wearer feel beautifully empowered.

Comfort is the key. It breeds confidence and positive emotions. Plant-based fabrics are a priority, especially because they are more comfortable than most synthetic apparel. If, at times, synthetic apparel is the only option, make sure synthetic garments are worn as the outer layers of an outfit, preferably not the first layer. Synthetic apparel is better when loose, not tight-fitting. Wear knit stretch fabrics. If the item of clothing is woven and stiff, make sure it's not constricting the body and there's enough space to move around in the garment.

Seeking out sleek, minimal design with fresh details keeps the look focused, yet appealing. Wearing a larger selection of colors can heal negative symptoms and balance the mind and body. Look for things that don't necessarily speak of fashion. The colors of a flower may inspire your next new color of choice in a garment. A color found in the woods or at the beach may signal comfort and sentimentality. Patterns, textures, and rhythmic sequence found within a look are virtually the "music" of fashion. Patterns create rhythm and movement within a design. They are visually and energetically stimulating. Patterns can literally set the tone for the day.

Layers are stylish and functional. They provide emotional and creative depth visually and literally within an outfit, creating balance within a look. Mix and match different types of styles together. A long tunic with boots paired with a bomber jacket. A trench coat with a hooded sweatshirt with a pair of leg warmers. This is about creating a universal look.

Playing with several fashion archetypes together creates more balance and universal fashion transparency; a style that's globally conscious. Mixing and matching different cultural pieces together gives an edge. Being able to take risks and not keep within the means of a specific, set look creates open-mindedness.

It helps to recognize fashion details like collars, necklines, hem lengths, colors, fabrics, and silhouettes that strengthen body features, while weakening the areas where attention doesn't want to be drawn. There are typically no rules. People of every age and of every shape or size can wear what they want. If it feels good, it looks good. What is flattering to someone is usually personal. Don't underestimate the power of trying something new. A garment that looks terrible on the rack may be your next staple piece.

Look to the streets. Street fashion is a source of inspiration. It gives off a feeling of renewal. It's fulfilling to walk and observe street style around a city or town, and see eye to eye with our external surroundings. Individual style is always of paramount importance. It's expressive and fun to stand out. Other times it feels easier to pare down a look, but this is not about fitting the part.

Making fashion collages with inspiring fashion magazine clippings can often mark new territory for a person's next statement piece, mood, or image to be declared in their wardrobe. It's therapeutic, sets a realm of inspiration, and it's a reflection of a person, a representation of their inner self.

Runway shows are sure to inspire. There's a story to tell through fashion, and fashion themes and stories are used to represent personality. Designers always engage a specific type of character, image, and personality, portraying an individual perspective.

Being modern is not always about what's currently selling. It's a curation of personal style while using cues of what's going on in the world to keep a look fresh. What *is* dated is if one is stuck in the past and doesn't want to change. This can show through one's clothing, but it may not even be about the clothing. It could be residual stuck energy from a stagnant time in one's life. Fashion moves. Bear in mind a sweater, for example, could be worn daily for a year, and if a person's attitude and mindset is changing, the sweater changes with the mindset, and it stays current.

Clothing that's in trend helps support modernity because it creates change. Looking modern, however, is not always demonstrated through trends alone. Karl Lagerfeld, renowned fashion designer, wore basically the same outfit in public for decades, yet he remained modern and fresh. It's not necessarily the clothes by themselves that make fashion modern. As Karl Lagerfeld said: "Fashion is an attitude more than a clothing detail."

Chapter 11

A Sustainable Future for Modern, Healthy Fashion Businesses

Eco fashion for human health

"Eco" stems from the word "ecology," which means the study and science of how people or organisms relate to each other or their environment. Additionally, eco fashion stands for a political movement to protect the environment. Eco fashion reflects the nature that surrounds us, creating a harmonious, balanced existence. Fashion needs to support both ecosystems — the environment and the human body — as we ourselves are mini eco-systems.

Currently, genetic engineering of crop plants is wreaking havoc on soils, causing crop and soil depletion. It diminishes the nutrients and health properties found in our food and plant fiber crops. Fashion waste systems are toxic, and fashion waste isn't decomposing at a healthy rate either. Synthetic fabric production is changing the Earth's oxygen levels. It's all about taking steps that will ultimately lead to a healthier lifestyle and planet.

There may be a pinnacle point in time when Earth becomes an oasis. If individuals take matters into their own hands, nurturing their surroundings and their own body, things will vastly improve. By eliminating the toxic realm of fashion, we create a healthier Earth. As humans evolve, the planet evolves.

A few aspects of what makes a fashion business ecological or sustainable:

Environmentally-friendly fashion waste disposal
In the USA alone, an average of 26 billion pounds of apparel

end up in the landfill per year.

There's a tool and evaluation process called Waste Hierarchy, in Europe, that helps protect the environment. To set priorities for waste management, they have a five-tiered framework: "Prevention, Reuse, Recycle, Recovery, Disposal."

The first step of the five-tiered framework takes preventative measures that adhere to sustainability practices and natural materials. In the reuse step, they find ways to give products a longer life cycle, and turn them over to shops that can assemble reused items. The recovery and disposal step is when they decipher if a waste product can be incinerated or disposed of in a landfill site. Incineration is a thermal treatment that turns the materials into ash, creating less waste. Pyrolysis and gasification are other solutions for trash disposal. Synthetic fabrics aren't suitable to be burned or incinerated, however, as they release dangerous, toxic chemicals into the air.

Burning large batches of tossed plant-based clothing and plant-based fashion waste is a great way to minimize landfill use. It is healthy to burn natural fibers. It was actually a sacred ritual to do so, in Israel. When plant-based fabrics are burned, they won't irritate humans, the air, or environment. Natural wildfires are considered healthy and are actually a benefit to the environment, so can burning 100% plant-based clothing. Additionally, Native Americans and other indigenous cultures burned plants like sage as a sacred ritual and in healing ceremonies to cleanse and purify themselves and the environment.

Commercial composting

Clothing in landfills is polluting the Earth and releasing toxic gases in the air, soil, and groundwater. Compostable fabrics reduce landfill use. Using clothing waste for compost can help foster new growth on the planet. A 100% plant-based fabric dyed with non-toxic dyes can be introduced back into the soil and composted.

If we had to look at a landfill nearby, we would think differently about trash. It's really out of sight out of mind. This is one reason it is so important for brands to incorporate a circular fashion model, and produce clothing that can be put back into the Earth on its last life cycle, where it will biodegrade and contribute to the planet in a healthy way.

If a garment is not suitable for thrift stores, or if a person doesn't want to shred their clothing and put it back into the land, there are large scale, commercial compost sites that will compost your natural clothing. A complete garment needs to be capable of breaking down into CO_2 within 180 days to be considered compostable.

Green delivery and retail packaging

Recycled, biodegradable and compostable packaging supports less waste in landfills and is less harmful to human and animal life. Instead of using petroleum-based plastic, biodegradable, biobased plastic packaging is an option. Recyclable and biodegradable hemp paper products are another option. In addition to hemp, sisal and jute fibers are an abundant resource and sustainable packaging material alternative. Using chlorine-free, unbleached paper packaging will help support the environment, especially the aquatic environment.

If printing on packaging is needed, soy, canola, safflower and linseed plant-based inks will make a package 100% biodegradable. They reduce carbon emissions, soil disruption, and so on. These vegetable-based inks can also be used for textile printing fabrics or direct to garment printing. Block, roller, screen, and heat transfer are a few textile printing methods.

Opting to produce reusable, high aesthetic, designer packaging is a branding strategy that encourages customer loyalty. Some designer packaging becomes a part of a fashion collector's storage, and is used and reused in various ways, while increasing its lifespan.

Green transportation: fashion product distribution and its carbon footprint

Based on the need for a healthier fashion industry, retailers and textile manufacturers distributing fair-trade fashion globally, while reducing their carbon footprint with environmentally-friendly green transportation, is a must. Product distribution involving green transportation is environmental, healthy, and natural. Global trade is important, but our carbon footprint can be a hazard due to carbon emissions from fossil fuel; especially when trains, trucks, and airplanes are not smog-tested and not eco-fueled. Eco certifications for trucks, planes, and boats that distribute fashion apparel are useful. Each industry is responsible for setting margins on how we are able to better support the environment.

Zero waste fashion

It is estimated that 15% of textiles are wasted from the fabric cutting process. Zero waste fashion pattern-making design technology for apparel manufacturing makes an effort to minimize the excess waste of leftover fabric scraps. Also, there are plenty of companies that take in these textile scraps that come from the pattern cutting phase of apparel production, for their resale.

Upcycled textiles

Textile upcycling is turning materials that are not fashion fabrics, like used garments, into another fashion fabric. Also, plant-based upcycling, such as turning paper products into fabrics and yarns, is healthy and a good recycling contribution.

Healthy fashion business strategies

In this section, I talk about several healthy fashion business practices. The fashion industry is vast. This section is not limited to speaking about fashion brands, but fashion businesses in general like: fashion retail, fashion show production, apparel manufacturing, fashion forecasting, and so on.

Management, strategy, and business development in fashion business plays a role. Yet the sole backbone of a fashion business is creativity and intuition. A company's story stems from creativity, and everything branches off from there. Creative inspiration and cultural life experiences can make or break a fashion business. Brands are extensions of personal and cultural beliefs. Part of a brand's strategy is to introduce lifestyle-based interests for their consumers, and express different lifestyles based on image, concept, vision, mission, and virtue.

Fashion brands or companies are influenced by RTW (ready-to-wear) and couture brands made with a strong theme and a creative, intuitive story, as their products are highlighted as "it" items. Inventive, modern brands and fashion businesses serve the community in the highest of light when their unique ideas are instilled, and when they are mindfully aware of their impact. Such a business has a strong, spiritual component to back up its message and product. They become a case of improving society compared with the soulless emptiness of some fashion businesses. Spiritless companies are based on wrong intentions. They won't prevail over the long haul.

Travel through books, film, or on foot, all are formal introductions to other worlds that broaden our view, and inspire us. The interconnection of art, music, and design fuels fashion. Other fields of study elevate fashion businesses by becoming foundation stones to help stabilize and support fashion ideas.

Merging and transcending conventional, eco/ sustainable, and healthy fashion together

Removing the barriers between conventional fashion, eco fashion, and healthy fashion is needed, on a grand scale. Eco fashion companies are involved in helping the environment. Those that are producing sustainable fabrics and fashions, they are most likely better equipped to produce healthy, medicinal fashion more quickly than mainstream fashion, because healthy fashion is relative to sustainable fashion.

Conventional, eco, and healthy fashion markets all need to feel included. Marketing and branding healthy fashion with words and terms like "whole," "holistic," "natural," and "plant-based," is much less guarding and more approachable for consumers and industry professionals that want to be a part of the scene.

Eco fashion is like a farm-to-table circuit revolving around its own course to some degree. However, eco fashion introduced in big retail sectors is in trend. For example, the large fashion brand, Aeropostale, had a whole line of recycled cotton garments as part of one of their seasonal collections, and they marketed them as eco fashion. Some larger retailers do promote eco fashion, usually in the form of capsule collections. This doesn't really cut it, because the select capsule-based product has limited availability.

Furthermore, style genres are limited within capsule collections. Capsule collections do not have the advantage of being made in multiple style genres for the unique needs of individuals. The mini, capsule collections may not vary enough in style due to the minimal range of product items produced. Additionally, even with the infiltration of sustainable products, conventional products usually crowd out the healthier products.

Infiltrating and merging healthy fashion within the larger scope of the fashion industry is a much more opportunistic and reliable method at this point than creating a rebellion against it and supporting a niche, eco fashion movement. It does influence, but eco fashion practice has to be reachable to all. Mainstream companies need to be motivated to participate, and feel they belong too. It's not about creating a niche, eco-culture against mainstream fashion. The solution is to treat healthy fashion like the way Whole Foods or Sprouts has treated food, becoming a mass chain supplier of healthy, alternative foods. Their strategy has worked, and it can be incorporated in fashion business.

Fashion is human-driven. It's a manmade act, down to the basics of needle, thread, and fabric. Fashion has to be created in order to be produced; therefore, it is our responsibility to create healthy or unhealthy fashion. Fashion that focuses on fixing oneself first is therefore a standard to be applied.

There's been somewhat of a block within the fashion industry that is preventing total environmental health from coming to fruition. Sustainable fashion is very concentrated on issues such as fixing the environment. However, if we look to the environment first in terms of fixing fashion for a healthier environment, we are misrepresenting our own human condition's basic need to put oneself first as a survival mechanism.

As we heal ourselves through fashion it then becomes a natural, healing method to treat the environment. Sustainable fashion serves to preserve the environment. Healthy fashion serves to preserve the human race. Choosing materials and designs to fix the body will have a more profoundly humane effect on both humanity and the environment.

When mainstream and eco fashion become healthier, this will open up new territory for healthy, medicinal fashion to come into play. Current sustainable strategies from all business industries in every field will influence each other, and they will eventually further extend their practices with matters of health included.

Authenticity in fashion businesses

Karl Lagerfeld, the former creative director and head designer of Chanel, is now deceased. He worked up to his death as the creative director for Chanel, maintaining the brand ever since the early 1980s up until his final show in 2019. Chanel may never again be as it was, with Coco Chanel and Karl Lagerfeld gone. The legacy of the brand will change, as it was clear he was a direct "voice" of the Chanel brand. Karl was a fashion intuitive for the brand. There might be new paths for Chanel as it embraces new impressions from the work of other designers, but very few people are intuitive fashion designers. Intuitive fashion designers can literally channel the spirit of a brand. So, there is a difference between a fashion designer and a fashion intuitive.

Chanel products will change as the destiny of many legacy brands partake in morphing them into something unclear to the original designer. Additionally, brands and major corporations can become conglomerates and become too big. They are no longer able to be controlled and different visions and intentions occur. The work then caters to something else, and the brands support an unnatural and artificial fashion industry. They are then no longer rooted in the original spirit of the brand. Brands may then become soulless and in pursuit of disingenuous intent; they simply form as a new entity of its own.

Transparency

Transparency in the supply chain is a major innovation and a future business standard for the fashion industry. The increased transparency of brands gives consumers much more control over their product choices. Transparency within a company also guarantees more workers' rights and ethical practices. Transparency in fashion creates business production guidelines that address fashion issues. This helps form a loyal partnership between businesses and their clients/customers, when they are allowed to get involved.

Fashion transparency allows consumers to navigate a company's supply chain, gaining insight into behind-the-scenes apparel manufacturing. When a company is transparent, and they answer questions customers have about fashion production, the consumers are able to address these issues themselves. Fashion transparency gives consumers access to how a garment is made, who made it, what it's made of, and where it was made. It creates consumer awareness, and helps to bring about an increase in ethical practice.

Some new apparel tracking systems are being developed, like digital fashion apps that can track products that are made with traceable product tags. A cellphone is used to scan an electronic product code usually printed on clothing tags. This tracking system provides the who, what, where, and how of a product to the customer. These navigational tools and programs that trace and reference information about a product are useful.

Transparency creates social awareness. It is sometimes thought-provoking to hear the story behind a purchased product. It's ultimately the responsibility of designers, brands, and fashion businesses to convey it. The research involved in sourcing ethical fashion takes time and energy. Fashion transparency made by fashion tech makes it easier and faster for the consumer.

The modern meaning of luxury fashion

Modern luxury fashion is not fashion that caters to the wealthy, and to those that are supposedly able to live in luxury because they own luxury goods. That's an outdated, very unwelcoming and discomforting way of perceiving luxury fashion for the greater population at large, and for those who can't afford or don't buy luxury goods. It should not be limited to high-priced fashions that only a small percentage can afford.

Modern luxury is defined here as something that expresses comfort and an increased awareness of comfort. It's not about the wealthy or high-class living. Fashion should be made a luxury to everyone, because luxurious living is about comfort, and we all need to be comforted by our fashions.

Luxury fashion for everyone

Luxury is a mood and a tone to be embraced by all. Healthy, luxury fashion creates a natural, ambient mood. When people perceive fashion as luxurious, they experience an emotional phenomenon. It is understood luxury goods evoke a sense of grace and ease. Luxury is an expression of trust, security, contentment, and confidence. These emotions are needed to be expressed and be a part of everyone's lifestyle in order to sustain wellbeing.

Luxury fashion is typically exclusive to the wealthy, and is often associated with pretentious people and businesses that support the idea that luxury is not something everyone can have. Pretentious people can give off a false representation of themselves, and act like they are superior to others because they can own luxury goods and can be in a state of luxury, and supposedly not everyone can have that. In this sense, luxury fashions are used as a weapon by pretentious people and corrupt companies, as they steal people's power in order to advance their own social status, career, or wealth.

Pretentiousness found in luxury fashion breeds a mindset fixed on false awareness. This dated fashion mentality is an ego-based idea of luxury, maintained by false power, contributing to the corruption and evil in the world. This is not a healthy fashion perception, and it doesn't contribute to equality.

Sometimes, people are fed the idea that if someone else can afford luxury goods they are more comfortably placed in society, and more comfortable in their own skin and luxury apparel. This is not a helpful perception, and it's an example of false programming, creating exclusion. This idea that only a select few get to purchase luxury goods needs to be modernized. Everyone needs luxury. Whether it be high or low fashion, luxury and comfort value need to be actualized through all sectors of the fashion markets with varying economic price points. Luxury is a mental attitude to be shared by all.

More and more, we will see brands contributing to a wider audience without reducing the luxury appeal of their products. People want luxury products because of their sentimental value. Investment pieces are likely chosen for their incredible style and aesthetic. Additionally, the higher prices of luxury goods do require consumers to think mindfully about their purchases and also make people want to take better care of them. A three hundred dollar jacket is going to get hung up, not crumpled up in the closet. So, this better care for clothes is an extension of treating ourselves better too. When we care for ourselves it's an act of luxury and it creates part of this "luxury attitude." We don't need expensive clothing to prompt us to take care of ourselves and our clothes more.

Luxury fashion is a lifestyle, an attitude, a mood, an alleviation, and can give a feeling of belonging. What makes a luxury brand successful is the quality and sentiment of the product. It is not only the price but also the intention and attention being put on the product to make it special and personal. The product then becomes emotionally sentimental. It is the style, design, and genuine meaning behind the garment that ultimately creates a sentimental attachment.

The concept of luxury needs to be a branding strategy in all fashion market platforms. Fashion luxury should be expressed through all low, medium and high fashion markets to balance out and freshen the economy and people's perception and their connection to fashion. While high-fashion, luxury apparel may be unaffordable to many, some lifestyle brands incorporate products available to every budget. It enhances their brand vision and mission while capitalizing on a lower price point. Yet, if we can't afford their luxury-based coats or pants, no one should have to buy a branded cosmetic item or a small purse in order to achieve a glimpse of luxury, that is just plain offensive. Yet, even still, these smaller priced products are an inspiration, and give people hope of that designer, branded dream, so it's not a bad thing.

Bottom line, however, is that a less wealthy person should feel just as luxurious in their outfits. There shouldn't be a fashion struggle in anyone's social class. There should be no interest of who gets to feel more luxurious in their wardrobe.

It is more important for high-fashion brands to design luxury fashion for multiple markets, rather than a high-fashion brand that can only give a customer a bottle of perfume or a keychain if they can't afford their clothing. We shouldn't have to spend thousands on a garment to enable it to be luxurious. That's why many high-fashion brands have contemporary to mid-level and mass-market collections along with their high-end label. Introducing luxury fashion through all designer, contemporary and mass fashion markets will bring positivity to consumers of all budgets. This can be easily accomplished through marketing, advertising, branding, and through fashion design and fashion business.

Slow fashion versus fast fashion

A leading conductor and cause of fast fashion is synthetic apparel. The production of fast fabrics produces fast fashion. With the industrial revolution came technologically induced machinery producing petroleum-based fabric. Less labor creates faster production turnover, leading to a perpetual cycle of faster, cheaper, and more. Plant crop cultivation for plant-based textiles takes its due course. Natural, organic textile production is a more natural, healthy production cycle and process, which will automatically slow down product consumption. Humans have a deeper connection with plants. We are less susceptible to throw it out as quickly as we throw out synthetic fabric fashions.

Some fast fashion brands' products appear to have less value because of their cheap factor. A lesser quality product is typically made in less time. Cheap, fast fashion apparel is mostly made with cheap fabrics, which cannot always withstand time, and many are synthetic or synthetically blended. This makes fast fashion affordable, and fits the budget-conscious mass market, making fast fashion an economic necessity.

The value of fast fashion products may be much less, yet because of its affordability, it's a popular trend as it provides for the lower to middle class which make up most of the population. Fast fashion can also be a matter of convenience, and this becomes a leading reason why people buy it. However, you can still buy fast fashion and incorporate it into a slow fashion, minimal-style wardrobe. This is still a sustainable fashion effort. Additionally, fast fashion can belong in all low, mid, and high markets. There's always a need for a mix of high, medium, and low fashion apparel, to create a healthy wardrobe.

Contemporary brands play an important role as middlemen between high and low fashion brands. Contemporary fashion merges and combines high and low fashion, and balances out slow and fast fashion. Slow fashion can be more expensive, offering higher-priced investment pieces. Typically, fast, throwaway fashion lives for no more than a few months to a few years, depending on usage. This can be due to its life cycle, damage, or because it is a fad item that doesn't stand the test of time. Bear in mind, a garment can also be moderately fast in production, yet can still be considered a "slow" garment.

The fashion industry is trend-driven, and it can still maintain trends and establish holistic cycles of fashion. Seasonal collections are here to promote personal and collective growth. Fast fashion trends that are produced with false intention can be materialistic, peer-influenced, and be influenced by corporate greed and social power. Endorsing healthier ways to produce a collection will enhance fashion looks, and these looks will prove to be interchangeable over time.

Fashion cycles can become exploited, but trends, in general, are naturally holistic. These cycles can be compared with a flower that develops from its seed, grows, blooms, then disintegrates in soil. In a similar way, a garment's life cycle withers and eventually dies from one's life. So, fashion is a catalyst of constant change and a tool for personal growth.

Trends are valuable in the way they can be holistic cycles that represent the times personally and collectively. Fashion will always move and grow along with the trends. Fashion moves like the natural flow and movement of nature's elements. The cycles of trends likened to the cycles of nature are virtually endless because fashion is in a constant state of evolution.

High fashion versus low fashion

Most high fashion is designer-made apparel. However, a low fashion garment with a high fashion aesthetic can still be called high fashion. Low fashion is typically based for the mass market. They are more simply made and cheaper and faster to make. Low fashion works for different lifestyle budgets, a reason it's popular, and highly accessible. High fashion does not lead consumer consumption or materialism, because it's made in smaller quantities, unless there's a constant need to purchase them because they are a part of a fad.

Accumulating too much of either high or low fashion in a

small amount of time, unless it's for a purpose, is not a healthy foundation for an individual, and it's hoarding. If one is a collector of fashion, that's different. Oftentimes, in the practice of minimalism, choosing to wear a smaller palette of garments creates a deeper human/fashion connection. Wearing dozens of different garments per month creates less attachment to them.

Consumers want options though, and that's a good thing. They don't always want to select a garment from a small closet of exclusive items, they desire variety. If low fashion is disposable, biodegradable, or burnable, it can make throwing clothing out not a drag, without it being a burden to the environment.

Throwaway, low fashion can be successful if it's compostable, plant-based, and can be fed back into land. It cannot hurt the environment, cause waste or deplete natural resources. Burning the clothing is even better. Huge toxic-fuming landfill piles are persisting. Synthetic fabric chemicals—toxic methane and carbon dioxide—are released into the air. Current throwaway fashion is mostly made from petroleum-based ingredients, which are top polluters. Synthetic-based fashion takes up to hundreds of years to biodegrade. They disrupt the soil and groundwater over the course of that time. A very large percentage of low fashion is made of synthetic materials or synthetic blends.

A higher-priced or higher-quality, high fashion garment provides an emotional sentiment. A high fashion brand and the personal sentiment of their products forms customer brand loyalty, and is a result of consumers wanting a high-quality, long-lasting garment with high designer aesthetic. If a garment is high fashion, that alone makes it more favorable and more likely to be worn. It's easier to throw away clothing containing pillage, stains, holes, or missing hardware like buttons and fasteners when price tags are low or the item was on sale.

However, many slow fashion garments can be considered high fashion, or of equivalent value, no matter its quality or aesthetic.

The presence behind a product, its style and charm, establishes a natural attraction and an inevitable attachment to a consumer. There is fair-priced fashion out there that satisfies such a sentiment. Some inexpensive items are well made, lasting many life cycles, becoming a major contribution to a person's life. This could be as simple as a tee shirt. A well-made, high fashion design can be as simple as a tee shirt, cheap and easy to make.

It takes cognition, insight, and technology to produce fashion that is more sustainable, and more socially and economically aware. Balancing high fashion and low fashion can support consumers of all budgets. Catering to different budgets, with an understanding of the importance of fashion reaching everyone, deliberately creates a healthier industry. When high fashion becomes low fashion, and vice versa, this will create a healthier fashion industry.

A Final Note

The information presented throughout the book has been vast, and with enough detail to fully capture the essence and the big picture of fashion's future. Fashion for health is a very intricate and complex operating force, and when fully integrated, it will yield promising results for all. Reviewing many of the possibilities healthy fashion has to offer, whether they are already practiced or not, this book makes sure to express the purpose and meaning behind fashion, very profoundly.

This extensive exploration into fashion in pursuit of health is not only a significant fashion forecast; it also makes a mark in the history of our evolution and where fashion is headed and where it is at present. Tapping into all of what *Healthy Fashion* offers, this is an opportunity for all of us.

Healthy Fashion really defines some of the major opportunities we have in order to revamp the current state of fashion. Reflecting on *Healthy Fashion* enables a person to enhance their own fashion insights for both personal and professional use.

More and more, fashion is a creative inspiration. The inspiration to transform our own wardrobes, our fashion industry, and be practitioners of healthy fashion is actualizing. We are part of a really exciting time for fashion.

Bibliography

Adelson, Cassandre/ Bordage, Ava/ Nunley, Jordan/ Parker, Kaitlyn (2019) "We Need a Nationwide Plastic Ban." [Online], *Debating Science Blog*, Umass.Edu Available at https://blogs.umass.edu/natsci397a-eross/we-need-a-nationwide-plastic-ban/ (Accessed November 2018)

Adgent, Margaret A./ Hoffman, Kate/ Goldman, Barbara D./ Sjödin, Andreas/ Daniels, Julie L. (2014) "Brominated Flame Retardants in Breast Milk and Behavioral and Cognitive Development at 36 Months." [Ejournal], *US National Library of Medicine*, National Institutes of Health. Available at https://www.ncbi.nlm.nih.gov/pmc/articles/PMC3997742/ (Accessed November 2018)

Agrawal, Bipin J. (2015) "Ayurvastra: Herbal fabrics designed for healing." [Ejournal], *Journal of Biotechnology & Biomaterials*, Omics International Conference Series. Available at https://www.omicsonline.org/proceedings/ayurvastra-herbal-fabrics-designed-for-healing-38977.html (Accessed October 2018)

Agricultural Outlook (1991) "Milkweed's Potential as Fiber and Filler." [Ebook], Agricultural Outlook, *The Service* (Accessed December 2018)

ArchaeoFeed (2017) "Evidence for plant dye of 3000-year-old textiles found." [Online], *ArchaeoFeed*. Available at https://archaeofeed.com/2017/07/evidence-for-plant-dye-of-3000-year-old-textiles-found/ (Accessed October 2018)

Archroma (n.d.) "EarthColors® by Archroma." [Online], Reinach, Switzerland, *Archroma*, UN Global Impact. Available at https://www.archroma.com/innovations/earth-colors-by-archroma (Accessed August 2018)

Ariel, Yisrael (n.d.) "Priestly Garments of the High Priests and the Ordinary Priests." [Online], Jerusalem, Israel, *The*

Temple Institute, International Department of the Temple Institute. Available at https://templeinstitute.org/priestly-garments/ (Accessed October 2018)

Ascension with the Ascended Masters (n.d.) "The Ascended Masters and the Ray Colours." [Online], New Zealand, *Ascension with the Ascended Masters*. Available at https://www.alphaimaging.co.nz/masters-and-the-ray-colours (Accessed October 2018)

Baily, Regina (2019) "The Structure and Function of a Cell Wall." [Online], New York, NY, *ThoughtCo*. Dot Dash Publishing Company. Available at https://www.thoughtco.com/cell-wall-373613 (Accessed October 2018)

Bhattacharya, Surajit (2012) "Wound Healing through the Ages." [Ejournal], Bethesda, MD, *National Center of Biotechnology*, US National Library of Medicine. Available at https://www.ncbi.nlm.nih.gov/pmc/articles/PMC3495363/ (Accessed September 2018)

Bilton, Nick (2015) "The Health Concerns in Wearable Tech" [Enewspaper], *The New York Times Company*. Available at https://www.nytimes.com/2015/03/19/style/could-wearable-computers-be-as-harmful-as-cigarettes.html (Accessed October 2018)

Blumberg, Naomi/ Ferry, Ellen (2019) "Oskar Schlemmer." [Online], Chicago, IL, *Britannica*, Encyclopedia Britannica. Available at https://www.britannica.com/biography/Oskar-Schlemmer (Accessed September 2018)

B-Orgon (n.d.) "How Does the Orgone Energy Affect Our Body and the Environment?" [Online], *B-Orgon*. Available at http://b-orgon.org/en/how-does-the-orgone-energy-affect-our-body/ (Accessed October 2018)

Buzea, Cristina/ Pacheco, Ivan I./ Robbie, Kevin (2008) "Nanomaterials and Nanoparticles: Sources and Toxicity." [Ejournal], *Research Gate*, Biointerphases. Available at https://www.researchgate.net/publication/301868634_

Nanomaterials_and_Nanoparticles_Sources_and_Toxicity (Accessed October 2018)

Callewaert, Chris/ De Maeseneire, Evelyn/ Kerckhof, Frederiek-Maarten, et al. (2014) "Microbial Odor Profile of Polyester and Cotton Clothes after a Fitness Session." [Ejournal], Ghent, Belgium, Flemish Government/Ghent University, *US National Library of Medicine*. American Society for Microbiology (ASM). Available at https://www.ncbi.nlm.nih.gov/pmc/articles/PMC4249026/ (Accessed May 2019)

Carocci, Max (2010) "Clad with the 'Hair of Trees': A History of Native American Spanish Moss Textile Industries." [Ejournal], *Academia*. Available at https://www.academia.edu/323417/Clad_With_theHair_of_Trees_A_History_of_Native_American_Spanish_Moss_Textile_Industries (Accessed January 2019)

CBAN (2013) "Genetically Modified Cotton." [Online], Ottawa, Canada, *Canadian Biotechnology Action Network*. Tides Canada. Available at https://cban.ca/gmos/products/on-the-market/cotton/genetically-modified-cotton-cban-factsheet/ (Accessed June 2018)

Chabad (n.d.) "Tekhelet: The Mystery of the Long-Lost Biblical Blue Thread." [Online], *Chabad Library*, Lubavitch World Headquarters. Available at https://www.chabad.org/library/article_cdo/aid/530127/jewish/Tekhelet-The-Mystery-of-the-Long-Lost-Biblical-Blue-Thread.htm (Accessed October 2018)

Chakma, Koushik/ Cicek, Nazim/ and Rahman, Mashiur (2017) "Fiber extraction efficiency, quality and characterization of cattail fibres for textile applications." [Ebook], *The Canadian Society for Bioengineering*. Available at http://www.csbe-scgab.ca/docs/meetings/2017/CSBE17025.pdf (Accessed November 2018)

Chanana, Bhawana/ Tanushree (n.d.) "Water Hyacinth: A Promising Textile Fibre Source." [Online], *Technical Textile*,

Fibre 2 Fashion. Available at https://www.technicaltextile. net/articles/water-hyacinth-a-promising-textile-fibre-source-7619 (Accessed January 2019)

Chen, J. (2015) "The History of Lyocell Rayon." [Ejournal], *Science Direct*, Elsevier B.V. Available at https://www. sciencedirect.com/topics/engineering/lyocell-fiber (Accessed July 2018)

Chhabra, Esha (2016) "The dirty secret about your clothes." [Enewspaper], *The Washington Post*. Available at https:// www.washingtonpost.com/business/the-dirty-secret-about-your-clothes/2016/12/30/715ed0e6-bb20-11e6-94ac-3d324840106c_story.html (Accessed October 2018)

Cole, Laura (2016) "Plant Life: the state of the world's plants." [Online], *Syon Geographical Ltd*, Syon Media. Available at https://geographical.co.uk/places/forests/item/1901-plant-life (Accessed October 2018)

Deyute (2014) "The 11 Benefits of jute fabrics that everyone should know." [Online], Alicante, Spain, *Deyute*. Available at https://www.deyute.com/sec/en/news/the-11-benefits-of-jute-fabrics-that-everyone-should-know/44 (Accessed November 2018)

DIP (2018) "Forest Wool—A Unique and Innovative Material." [Online], *Development in Practice*. Available at http://dip.ng/journal/2018/5/29/forest-wool-a-unique-and-innovative-material (Accessed December 2018)

Dusenbury, Mary (1992) "A Wisteria Grain Bag and other tree bast fiber textiles of Japan." [Online], *Textiles in Daily Life: Proceedings of the Third Biennial Symposium of the Textile Society of America*. Available at https://digitalcommons.unl. edu/tsaconf/569/ (Accessed January 2019)

Eco Watch (2015), "84,000 Chemicals on the Market, Only 1% Have Been Tested for Safety." [Online], *Eco Watch*. Available at https://www.google.com/amp/s/www.ecowatch.com/84-000-chemicals-on-the-market-only-1-have-been-tested-for-safety-1882062458.amp.html (Accessed November 2018)

Eichhorn, Steven (2009), "Banana Leaf Fiber." [Ebook], *Handbook of Textile Fibre Structure: Volume 2: Natural, Regenerated, Inorganic and Specialist Fibres*, Elsevier. (Accessed November 2018)

Encyclopedia Britannica (2019) "Hemp: Plant." [Online], Chicago, IL, *Britannica*. Available at https://www.britannica.com/plant/hemp (Accessed November 2018)

Envirotextile (n.d.) "Agave Fiber Products." [Online], *Envirotextiles LLC*. Available at https://www.envirotextile.com/agave-fiber-products/ (Accessed November 2018)

Ettitude (2019) "Not All Bamboo Sheets Are Created Equal." [Online]. Available at https://ettitude.com/fabrics/not-bamboo-sheets-created-equal/ (Accessed November 2018)

Fibre 2 Fashion (2014) "Textiles made from Agave fibres." [Online], *Fibre 2 Fashion Pvt. Ltd*. Available at https://www.fibre2fashion.com/industry-article/7302/textiles-made-from-agave-fibres (Accessed November 2018)

Finkel, Joe/ James, Ruby/ Miller, Herbert (1979) "Residual Monomers in Acrylic and Modacrylic Fibers and Fabrics: Final Report." [Ebook], Washington, D.C., Office of Toxic Substances, United States Environmental Protection Agency. Available at https://nepis.epa.gov/Exe/ZyPURL.cgi?Dockey=9101AM9F.TXT (Accessed November 2018)

Fraunhofer-Gesellschaft (2013) "Using cattails for insulation." [Online], Rockville, MD, *Science Daily*. Available at https://www.sciencedaily.com/releases/2013/06/130603091730.htm (Accessed November 2018)

Future Fibers (n.d.) "Coir." [Online], *Food and Agriculture Organization of the United Nations*. Available at http://www.fao.org/economic/futurefibres/fibres/coir/en/ (Accessed November 2018)

Galang, Elson Ian Nyl (2012) "Eco-fabric from Blended Fragrant Screw Pine (Pandanus amaryllifolius) Leaf Fibers and

Cotton." [Ejournal], *Conference: Intel International Science and Engineering Fair*, Research Gate. Available at https://www. researchgate.net/publication/330135634_Eco-fabric_from_ Blended_Fragrant_Screw_Pine_Pandanus_amaryllifolius_ Leaf_Fibers_and_Cotton (Accessed December 2018)

Gant, James (2019) "A crude awakening: Bathing in oil is touted as health cure in Azerbaijan spa—despite doctors warning it could give you cancer." [Enewspaper], *Daily Mail UK*. Available at https://www.google.com/amp/s/www. dailymail.co.uk/news/article-6915873/amp/Azerbaijan- oil-baths-touted-health-cure-despite-doctors-warning- CANCER.html (Accessed November 2018)

Garb, Nitan (2010) "Study of Ramie Fibre—A Review." [Online], *Fibre 2 Fashion Pvt. Ltd.* Available at https://www. fibre2fashion.com/industry-article/4787/study-of-ramie- fibre-a-review (Accessed January 2019)

Goldberg, Eleanor (2016) "You're Probably Going to Throw Away 81 Pounds of Clothing This Year." [Enewspaper], New York, NY, *HuffPost News*. Available at https://www. huffpost.com/entry/youre-likely-going-to-throw-away-81- pounds-of-clothing-this-year_n_57572bc8e4b08f74f6c069d3 (Accessed October 2018)

Goodman, Sara/ Garcia, Michel/ Ingram, William (2013) "The Plant Mordant Project." [Ebook], Bali, Indonesia, *Bebali Foundation*. Available at http://box19.ca/maiwa/pdf/ symplocos.pdf (Accessed October 2018)

Graham, Helen (1998) "Color Therapy in the Ancient World and Middle Ages." [Online], Berkeley, CA, *Inner Self*, "Discover Color Therapy: A First-Step Handbook to Better Health," Ulysses Press. Available at https://innerself.com/ content/living/health/healing-disciplines/4639-color- therapy-through-the-ages-by-helen-graham.html (Accessed September 2018)

Hickey, Hannah (2008) "Toxic chemicals found in common

scented laundry products, air fresheners." [Online], *UW News*, University of Washington. Available at https://www.washington.edu/news/2008/07/23/toxic-chemicals-found-in-common-scented-laundry-products-air-fresheners/ (Accessed October 2018)

IARC (2004) "IARC Classifies Formaldehyde as Carcinogenic." [Online], *Oncology Times*, Wolters Kluwer Health. Available at https://journals.lww.com/oncology-times/full text/2004/07100/IARC_Classifies_Formaldehyde_as_Carcinogenic.27.aspx (Accessed November 2018)

Ibrahim, W./ Sarwar, Z./ Abid, S./ Munir, U./ Azeem, A. (2017) "Aloe Vera Leaf Gel Extract for Antibacterial and Softness Properties of Cotton." [Ejournal], *Journal of Textile Science & Engineering*. Available at https://www.hilarispublisher.com/open-access/aloe-vera-leaf-gel-extract-for-antibacterial-and-softness-properties-ofcotton-2165-8064-1000301.pdf (Accessed November 2018)

Indohemp (2019) "Hemp Material Benefits: 20 Great Facts About Hemp Fiber." [Online], *Indohemp*. Available at https://indohemp.com/blog/hemp-material-benefits/ (Accessed November 2018)

Intagliata, Christopher (2014) "Synthetic Fabrics Host More Stench-Producing Bacteria." [Online], *Scientific American*, Springer Nature America Inc. Available at https://www.scientificamerican.com/podcast/episode/synthetic-fabrics-host-more-stench-producing-bacteria/ (Accessed May 2018)

Jones, Jonathan (2016) "A human skin handbag is not fashion — it's a crime." [Enewspaper], New York, NY, *The Guardian*. Available at https://www.theguardian.com/artanddesign/jonathanjonesblog/2016/jul/19/alexander-mcqueen-human-skin-handbag-tina-gorjanc (Accessed November 2018)

Journal Star (2004) "Scientist uses cornhusks to develop textile fibers." [Online], Lincoln, NE, *Lincoln Journal Star*. Available at https://journalstar.com/news/state-and-regional/nebra

ska/scientist-uses-cornhusks-to-develop-textile-fibers/
article_716ac03e-e5a7-5d4f-b57d-cc491da8fead.html
(Accessed November 2018)

Kennedy, Wendy (n.d.) "What Exactly Are Galactic Light Codes?" [OU Module], *Higher Frequencies*. Available at https://galacticlightcodes.net (Accessed October 2018)

King, Godfrey R. (1993) *The Magic Presence* [Book], Schaumburg, IL, Saint Germain Press (Accessed October 2018)

Koca, Ozlem/ Altoparlak, Ulku/ Ayyildiz, Ahmet/ Kaynar, Hasan (2012) "Persistence of Nosocomial Pathogens on Various Fabrics." [Ejournal], Erzurum, Turkey, *Department of Microbiology and Clinical Microbiology*, Ataturk University, National Center for Biotechnology Information. Available at https://www.ncbi.nlm.nih.gov/pmc/articles/PMC4261405/ (Accessed November 2018)

Lafferty, Mike (2010) "Keeping up with detergent chemistry." [Online], *The American Oil Chemists' Society*, AOCS. Available at https://www.aocs.org/stay-informed/inform-magazine/featured-articles/keeping-up-with-detergent-chemistry-august-2010 (Accessed October 2018)

Lankston, Louise/ Cusack, Pearce/ Fremantle, Chris/ Isles, Chris (2010) "Visual art in hospitals: case studies and review of the evidence." [Ejournal], Greater Glasgow and Clyde, UK, *National Institute of Health*, Journal of the Royal Society of Medicine. Available at https://www.ncbi.nlm.nih.gov/pmc/articles/PMC2996524/ (Accessed September 2018)

Lenzing Aktiengesellschaft (2017) "Tencel—The New Age Fiber." [Ebook], Lenzing, Australia, *Lenzing Group*. Available at http://soluttions.com/wp-content/uploads/2016/12/pdf-Tencel_Folder_110717_screen1.pdf

Lymbery, Philip (2017) "Strategic Plan 2013–2017: For Kinder, Fairer Farming Worldwide." [Ebook], Surrey, UK, *Compassion in World Farming*. Available at https://www.ciwf.org.uk/media/3640540/ciwf_strategic_plan_20132017.

pdf (Accessed November 2018)

MacDonald, Matthew (2009) " Skin: Your Outer Layer." [OU Module], Boston, MA, *Your Body, The Missing Manual*, O'Reilly Media Inc. Available at https://www.oreilly.com/library/view/your-body-the/9780596805456/ch01.html (Accessed August 2018)

Mahapatra, N. N. (2017) "Clothing made from pineapple fiber." [Online], *Textile Today*. Available at https://www.textiletoday.com.bd/clothing-made-pineapple-fiber/ (Accessed October 2018)

Markowitz, Gerald/ Rosner, David (2018) "Monsanto, PCBs, and the creation of a 'world-wide ecological problem.'" [Ejournal], *Springer Link*, Springer Nature Switzerland AG. Available at https://link.springer.com/article/10.1057/s41271-018-0146-8 (Accessed November 2018)

Mazar, Anne (2014) "Down to Earth: Concerns about 80,000 Chemicals." [Online], Beverly, MA, *Wicked Local Salem*, Gannett Media Corp. Available at https://salem.wickedlocal.com/article/20140502/entertainmentlife/140509198 (Accessed October 2018)

Monatomic Orme (n.d.) "Monatomics." [Online], Ilderton, Canada. Available at https://monatomic-orme.com/about-orme/ (Accessed October 2018)

Morgan, Stuart (n.d.) "The boots that helped conquer Everest." [Online], *Satra Technology Centre*. Available at https://www.satra.com/bulletin/article.php?id=1067 (Accessed November 2018)

Murai, Tatsuhiko/ Murai, Ryoko (2014) "Changing of Kudzu Textiles in the Japanese Culture." *[Ebook]*, *Textile Society of American Symposium Proceedings*, University of Nebraska, Lincoln. Available at https://digitalcommons.unl.edu/cgi/viewcontent.cgi?article=1916&context=tsaconf (Accessed November 2018)

Natural Chakra Healing (n.d.) "Color as Energy

Nutrition." *Natural Chakra Healing*. Available at https://naturalchakrahealing.com/color-therapy.html (Accessed September 2018)

NBC News (2007) "Medical Microchip for People May Cause Cancer." [Online], *NBC News* Associated Press. Available at http://www.nbcnews.com/id/20643620/ns/health-cancer/t/medical-microchip-people-may-cause-cancer/#.XjdpX47Y-r8k (Accessed October 2018)

Neill, Conor (2018) "Understanding Personality: The 12 Jungian Archetypes." [Online], *Conor Neill*, Vistage. Available at: https://www.google.com/amp/s/conorneill.com/2018/04/21/understanding-personality-the-12-jungian-archetypes/amp/ (Accessed September 2018)

New York Times (1991) "Science Watch; The Nylon Effect." [Enewspaper], *The New York Times*. Available at https://www.nytimes.com/1991/02/26/science/science-watch-the-nylon-effect.html (Accessed November 2018)

Oceanic Institute (n.d.) "Aqua Facts." [Online], Waimanalo, HI. *Oceanic Institute*, Hawaii Pacific Ocean University. Available at https://www.oceanicinstitute.org/aboutoceans/aquafacts.html (Accessed July 2018)

Ort, Victoria (2006) "Skin and Sensory Receptors." [Online], *Education Med*, New York University NYU, Medical Center. Available at http://education.med.nyu.edu/Histology/coursematerials/syllabus/Skin.html (Accessed August 2018)

Paddison, Laura (2016) "Single clothes wash may release 700,000 microplastic fibres, study finds." [Enewspaper], New York, NY, *The Guardian*. Available at https://www.theguardian.com/science/2016/sep/27/washing-clothes-releases-water-polluting-fibres-study-finds (Accessed October 2018)

Pearsall, Paul P. (1999) "The Cellular Symphony." [Ebook], *The Heart's Code: Tapping the Wisdom and Power of Our Heart Energy*, Potter Ten. (Accessed October 2018)

Pere'rah, Rodney (2011) "The Power of Linen." [Online], *New*

2 *Torah*. Available at http://www.new2torah.com/2011/11/the-power-of-linen/ (Accessed September 2018)

Pickering, Kim (2008) "Natural Fibers: Types and Properties." [Ebook], *Properties and Performance of Natural-Fibre Composites*, Elsevier. (Accessed October 2018)

Rehan, Kelly/ Erickson, Karen (2019) "How Fashion Ergonomics Helps Your Spine." [Online], *Spine Universe*, Remedy Health Media. Available at https://www.google.com/amp/s/www.spineuniverse.com/amp/47832 (Accessed August 2018)

RFID Journal (2010) "Animal RFID Chip Implants Linked to Cancer." [Online], *RFID Journal*, Haycco. Available at https://www.rfidjournal.com/articles/view?6817 (Accessed October 2018)

Sageshima, Makiko / Takashima, Mami / Shirai, Fumie / Ikeda, Nanae / Shirai, Fumie (2004) "Distinctive bacteria-binding property of cloth materials." [Online], *American Journal of Infection Control*, Pub Med. Available at Research Gate (Access November 2018)

Samatoa Lotus Farm. "Lotus Fabric: The Most Spiritual Fabric." [Online], Siem Reap, Cambodia, *Samatoa*. Available at https://samatoa.lotus-flower-fabric.com/eco-textile-mill/lotus-fabric/?v=7516fd43adaa (Accessed December 2018)

Sasawashi (n.d.) "Concept." [Online], *Sasawashi*. Available at http://sasawashi.com/en/about/ (Accessed January 2019)

Science Learning Hub, Pokapu Akoranga Putaiao (n.d.) "Wool Fibre Properties." [Online], Hamilton, New Zealand, *Curious Minds*. Available at https://www.sciencelearn.org.nz/resources/875-wool-fibre-properties (Accessed November 2018)

Seido Japan (2017) "Aizome—Japanese Indigo on Martial Arts Equipment." [Online], Wako-shi, Shirako, *Seido Shop*. Available at https://www.seidoshop.com/blogs/the-seido-blog/44-aizome-japanese-indigo-on-budo-equipment (Accessed October 2018)

Shaari, Nazlina (2006) "Lemba (Curculigo latifolia) Leaf as a New Materials for Textiles." *Environmentally Conscious Design and Inverse Manufacturing*, Research Gate. Available at https://www.researchgate.net/publication/4235631_Lemba_Curculigo_latifolia_Leaf_as_a_New_Materials_for_Textiles

Shankman, Sabrina (2019) "What Is Nitrous Oxide and Why Is It a Climate Threat?" [Online], *Inside Climate News*. Available at https://insideclimatenews.org/news/11092019/nitrous-oxide-climate-pollutant-explainer-greenhouse-gas-agriculture-livestock (Accessed November 2018)

Smart Fiber Ag (n.d.) "SeaCell™ MT—Modal technology brings the power of seaweed to a fiber." [Ebook], *Smart Fiber Ag*. Available at https://www.smartfiber.de/en/fibers/seacelltm/ (Accessed January 2019)

Srivastava, Nupur/ Rastogi, Deepali (2018) "Nettle fiber: Himalayan wonder with extraordinary textile properties." [Ejournal], *International Journal of Home Science*. Available at http://www.homesciencejournal.com/archives/2018/vol4issue1/PartE/4-1-57-662.pdf (Accessed December 2018)

SSRF (n.d.) "Spiritual Properties of Cotton Cloth and Clothes Made from Cotton." [Online], *Spiritual Science Research Foundation Inc.* Available at https://www.spiritualresearchfoundation.org/spiritual-living/how-to-dress/spiritual-properties-cotton-cloth/ (Accessed October 2018)

St. Clair, Kassia (2017) "The Secret Lives of Colors" [Ebook], *Penguin*. (Accessed October 2018)

Tarver-Wahlquist, Sarah/ Fernandez Rysavy, Tracy/ Floyd, André (n.d.) "The Trouble with Nano-Fabrics." [Online], *Green America*. Available at https://www.greenamerica.org/detox-your-closet-search-less-toxic-clothes/trouble-nano-fabrics (Accessed October 2018)

Teague, Lynn S. (1999) "Textiles and Prehistory." [Ebook],

Arizona State Museum, *Archaeology Southwest Magazine.* Available at https://www.archaeologysouthwest.org/pdf/ arch-sw-v13-no4.pdf (Accessed October 2018)

Turgeon, Andrew (2018) "Petroleum." [Online], *National Geographic.* National Geographic Society. Available at https://www.nationalgeographic.org/encyclopedia/ petroleum/ (Accessed July 2018)

United Nations (2004) "Pesticide poisoning affects children at higher rate—UN agencies." [Online], *UN News.* Available at https://news.un.org/en/story/2004/10/117052-pesticide- poisoning-affects-children-higher-rate-un-agencies (Accessed October 2018)

University of British Columbia (n.d.) "Lecture 6, Cellulose Chemistry." [OU Module], Vancouver, British Columbia, *Course Hero Inc.* Available at https://www.coursehero. com/file/37121680/Lecture6CelluloseChemistrypptx-4pdf/ (Accessed August 2018)

Ventura-Camargo, Bruna de Campos/ Marin-Morales, Maria Aparecida (2013) "Azo Dyes: Characterization and Toxicity—A Review." [Ejournal], *Research Gate,* Textile and Light Industrial Science and Technology. Available at https://www.researchgate.net/publication/282815745_ Azo_Dyes_Characterization_and_Toxicity-_A_Review (Accessed November 2018)

Wikipedia (2020) "Beauty and cosmetics in ancient Egypt." [Online], *Wikipedia, The Free Encyclopedia.* Available at https://en.wikipedia.org/wiki/Beauty_and_cosmetics_in_ ancient_Egypt (Accessed October 2018)

Wikipedia (2016) "BioSteel." [Online], *Wikipedia, The Free Encyclopedia.* Available at https://en.wikipedia.org/wiki/ BioSteel (Accessed November 2018)

Wikipedia (2020) "Bt Cotton." [Online], *Wikipedia, The Free Encyclopedia.* Available at https://en.wikipedia.org/wiki/ Bt_cotton (Accessed November 2018)

Wikipedia (2019) "Category: Fashion Aesthetics." [Online], *Wikipedia, The Free Encyclopedia.* Available at https://en.wikipedia.org/wiki/Category:Fashion_aesthetics (Accessed September 2018)

Wikipedia (2020) "Composition of the human body." [Online], *Wikipedia, The Free Encyclopedia.* Available at https://en.m.wikipedia.org/wiki/Composition_of_the_human_body (Accessed July 2018)

Wikipedia (2019) "Pina." [Online], *Wikipedia, The Free Encyclopedia.* Available at: https://en.wikipedia.org/wiki/Pi%C3%B1a (Accessed December 2018)

Wikipedia (2020) "Timeline of Monsanto." [Online], *Wikipedia, The Free Encyclopedia.* Available at https://en.wikipedia.org/wiki/Timeline_of_Monsanto (Accessed August 2018)

Woodford, Chris (2019) "Piezoelectricity." [Online], *Explain That Stuff.* Available at https://www.explainthatstuff.com/piezoelectricity.html (Accessed September 2018)

Wilinger, Gunther (2016) "The aluminium trees of Sulawesi." [Online], *Institute for Systematic Botany and Ecology,* Bioeconomy BW. Available at https://www.biooekonomie-bw.de/en/articles/news/the-aluminium-trees-of-sulawesi (Accessed October 2018)

Williams, Randy (n.d.) "Red Dirt Shirts Faqs" [Online], Eleele, Hawaii, Original Red Dirt Shirts™. Available at http://dirtshirt.com/index.php?route=information/information&information_id=8 (Accessed October 2018)

Zyga, Lisa (2010) "Scientists breed goats that produce spider silk." [Online], *Phys Org,* Science X Network. Available at https://phys.org/news/2010-05-scientists-goats-spider-silk.html (Accessed November 2018)

About the Author

Alyssa Couture is an author, fashion designer, and fashion entrepreneur. She is currently focused on her fresh-inspired Healthy Fashion Campaign, which is in conjunction with her book: *Healthy Fashion.*

Alyssa is a fashion industry expert, with over 15 years' fashion industry experience in a number of roles. Some of which include: fashion business, fashion designing, creative directing, styling, merchandising, fashion journalism, fashion retailing, and fashion show production.

Apart from fashion, she has a spiritually driven lifestyle, having previously lived in several ashrams and monasteries. She is a professional fine artist/illustrator with published and sold works to follow. She is a major foodie and former chef claiming 5 Star reviews.

Alyssa has lived and worked in NH, NYC, New Jersey, West Virginia, Michigan, and in her most favored and current location: California. Her love of travel has given her the opportunity to explore different cultures and influence her outlook.

Alyssa is a fashion intuitive. Her sole motive is to bring fashion into its course as a modern, therapeutic, healing tool. Her work involves initiating the consciousness of the human spirit via fashion, into its transmission of divine activity for overall human health and wellbeing, and for the ultimate planetary awakening.

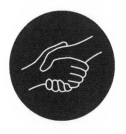

AYNI
BOOKS

ALTERNATIVE HEALTH & HEALING

"Ayni" is a Quechua word meaning "reciprocity" - sharing, giving and receiving - whatever you give out comes back to you. To be in Ayni is to be in balance, harmony and right relationship with oneself and nature, of which we are all an intrinsic part. Complementary and Alternative approaches to health and well-being essentially follow a holistic model, within which one is given support and encouragement to move towards a state of balance, true health and wholeness, ultimately leading to the awareness of one's unique place in the Universal jigsaw of life - Ayni, in fact. If you have enjoyed this book, why not tell other readers by posting a review on your preferred book site.

Recent bestsellers from AYNI Books are:

Reclaiming Yourself from Binge Eating
A Step-By-Step Guide to Healing
Leora Fulvio, MFT
Win the war against binge eating, wake up each morning at peace with your body, unafraid of food and overeating.
Paperback: 978-1-78099-680-6 ebook: 978-1-78099-681-3

The Reiki Sourcebook (revised ed.)
Frans Stiene, Bronwen Stiene
A popular, comprehensive and updated manual for the Reiki novice, teacher and general reader.
Paperback: 978-1-84694-181-8 ebook: 978-1-84694-648-6

The Chakras Made Easy
Hilary H. Carter
From the successful Made Easy series, Chakras Made Easy is a practical guide to healing the seven chakras.
Paperback: 978-1-78099-515-1 ebook: 978-1-78099-516-8

The Inner Heart of Reiki
Rediscovering Your True Self
Frans Stiene
A unique journey into the inner heart of the system of Reiki, to help practitioners and teachers rediscover their True Selves.
Paperback: 978-1-78535-055-9 ebook: 978-1-78535-056-6

Middle Age Beauty
Soulful Secrets from a Former Face Model Living Botox Free in her Forties
Machel Shull
Find out how to look fabulous during middle age without plastic surgery by learning inside secrets from a former model.
Paperback: 978-1-78099-574-8 ebook: 978-1-78099-575-5

The Optimized Woman
Using Your Menstrual Cycle to Achieve Success and Fulfillment
Miranda Gray
If you want to get ahead, get a cycle! For women who want to create life-success in a female way.
Paperback: 978-1-84694-198-6

The Patient in Room Nine Says He's God
Louis Profeta
A roller coaster ride of joy, controversy, triumph and tragedy;
often all on the same page.
Paperback: 978-1-84694-354-6 ebook: 978-1-78099-736-0

Re-humanizing Medicine
A Holistic Framework for Transforming Your Self, Your Practice,
and the Culture of Medicine
David Raymond Kopacz
Re-humanizing medical practice for doctors, clinicians, clients, and
systems.
Paperback: 978-1-78279-075-4 ebook: 978-1-78279-074-7

**You Can Beat Lung Cancer Using Alternative/Integrative
Interventions**
Carl O. Helvie R.N., Dr.P.H.
Significantly increase your chances of long-term lung cancer
survival by using holistic alternative and integrative interventions
by physicians or health practitioners.
Paperback: 978-1-78099-283-9 ebook: 978-1-78099-284-6

Readers of ebooks can buy or view any of these bestsellers by
clicking on the live link in the title. Most titles are published in
paperback and as an ebook. Paperbacks are available in traditional
bookshops. Both print and ebook formats are available online.

Find more titles and sign up to our readers' newsletter at http://
www.johnhuntpublishing.com/mind-body-spirit
Follow us on Facebook at https://www.facebook.com/OBooks and
Twitter at https://twitter.com/obooks